# A BUMP IN THE ROAD

# A BUMP IN THE ROAD

MY MEDICAL JOURNEY OVER
POTHOLES, DETOURS, AND
THE BRIDGE TO GRATITUDE

MICHAEL CAPRIO

NEW DEGREE PRESS

A BUMP IN THE ROAD

*My Medical Journey over Potholes, Detours, and the Bridge to Gratitude*

| ISBN | | |
|---|---|---|
| | 978-1-63676-362-0 | *Hardback* |
| | 978-1-63676-850-2 | *Paperback* |
| | 978-1-63730-192-0 | *Kindle Ebook* |
| | 978-1-63730-294-1 | *Ebook* |

"*The longer I live, the more I realize the impact of attitude on life. Attitude, to me, is more important than facts. It is more important than the past, than education, than money, than circumstances, than failures, than successes, than what other people think or say or do. It is more important than appearance, giftedness, or skill. It will make or break a company. . . a church. . . a home. The remarkable thing is we have a choice every day regarding the attitude we will embrace for that day. We cannot change our past. . . we cannot change the fact that people will act in a certain way. We cannot change the inevitable. The only thing we can do is play on the one string we have, and that is our attitude. . . I am convinced that life is 10% what happens to me and 90% how I react to it. And so it is with you. . . we are in charge of our attitudes.*"

—CHARLES SWINDOLL

# CONTENTS

_____

*In loving memory of my grandparents Donald and Juanita McGraw.*

*Without your support and guidance, this would have never been possible. What was once a silly idea I was too insecure to talk about is now officially a reality. You guys always encouraged me to chase my dreams and always believed in my abilities. Gram, without you I would've never been open enough to share this journey. Hearing all your stories of perseverance and how you talked about it with such humility inspired me to do the same. Pop, your values of hard work taught me to keep pushing through the difficult times. You taught me to believe in myself and to be strong. They say it takes a village to raise a child, and I had the best, most loving village I could've ever asked for. Your values, morals and lessons that were taught to me molded me into the man I am today. I know how much this meant to my grandma specifically because of the condition we share. Our story is finally public, Gram, and I hope it has the impact we thought it could have.*

# INTRODUCTION

———

In life, they say there are moments so overwhelming that time physically screeches to a halt. Events moving at a break-neck pace slow down like you've entered some crazy version of *The Matrix*. This is your body entering "fight or flight." When you enter this dimension, you perceive the threat viscerally and everything around you truly goes in slow motion, likely in an effort to make optimal survival decisions. Sounds like something corny out of a science-fiction movie, but I can assure you this isn't bullshit.

I can remember the first time in my life that I entered this matrix and the first time I felt my protective shield of childhood ignorance get obliterated by life's unpredictable nature. The only problem for me when I entered the matrix was that I *wasn't* running from a bear, getting mugged, or swerving my car to avoid a potentially fatal accident. Instead, I was being strapped onto an ice-cold operating table in a metallic room that bounced the light off every corner of my four-dimensional hell.

I was a terrified, immature, eighteen year old getting his first dose of the scary challenges life can throw at you. A team of medical personnel strapped me into place on the blistering cold surface. Goosebumps dotted my skin up and down my body as my hair stood straight up like it was standing at attention, waiting to be relieved of its duties. Perhaps it wasn't that cold, and maybe it was my nerves causing me to shake like I had just undergone Navy SEALs training. Whatever the cause of my shaking, I was officially entering uncharted territory. I analyzed the room while doctors and nurses worked in slow motion strapping my arms into place.

*No turning back now!*

I couldn't move to break free if I wanted to, but I continued to observe my surroundings as my inevitable fate trudged its way toward me. This date with destiny wasn't going to be postponed, and I certainly couldn't run away from this battle.

Once I was secured, I watched the nurse on my right slide a table full of scalpels, knives, and other sterile shiny objects that were going to be used to cut me open. The severity of the situation began to dawn on me, and my heart rate increased.

*Bud-um, bud-um, bud-um.*

Sweat dripped down my forehead and my back as it crystallized to the cold surface, adding to my agony. I stared at the medical team for what felt like an eternity (in reality, it was probably only a couple of minutes). The doctor on my right put the oxygen mask over my nose and mouth. The gas irritated my nostrils as the anesthesia shot up my arm on its way to my brain. I took in my last seconds of consciousness. When I woke up, my world would be completely different. I tried to savor what could have been the last seconds of my life here on this planet. Then, darkness...

The date was July 10 when I had my first of two lifesaving operations. I was under the knife for nine hours on that day to get the entirety of my large intestine removed. Sounds dramatic, but this is what happens when you're diagnosed with familial adenomatous polyposis. I know it's a chore to pronounce or read that name over and over again, so we'll stick to calling it FAP for short.

FAP is a rare, inherited condition caused by a defect in the adenomatous polyposis coli (APC) gene.[1] In short, what that means is that my body causes extra tissue or polyps to multiply and grow in my large intestine.[2] With my condition, there is no "if" that I will get cancer, but "when." FAP patients typically don't see cancer until their forties, but it will show up sometimes sooner.[3] I can say with a great deal of confidence that if I didn't get operated on at eighteen, I would be severely sick by now or possibly dead, as my colonoscopy revealed hundreds if not thousands of polyps growing in my large intestine.

Thus, I was introduced to the world of being a medical anomaly, experiencing things a select few go through. FAP affects only one in five to ten thousand Americans per year and accounts for 0.5 percent of all cases of colorectal cancer.[4] According to national registries, that is just 2.29 to 3.2 per 100,000 individuals.[5] So, it's safe to say I'm a needle in the haystack when it comes to medical conditions. That's a feeling that can plague an emotionally immature, naive teenager like myself, and it sure did.

---

1    "Familial Adenomatous Polyposis," Mayo Clinic, Mayo Foundation for Medical Education and Research, December 21, 2018.

2    Ibid.

3    Ibid.

4    "Familial Adenomatous Polyposis," NORD (National Organization for Rare Disorders), Accessed January 8, 2021.

5    Ibid.

Eighteen is a confusing age to begin with, and I was especially lost. The normal stuff that occupies space in your mind when you're a senior in high school, like fitting in with certain cliques, dealing with bullies, and deciding what I wanted to do with my life, became an exponentially more complicated equation once I got diagnosed. *How can you even focus on what you want to do with your life when you don't know what your life is going to be like next year?*

That's the first time I was introduced to the outsider, as I've dubbed it: that annoying voice in your head that tells you you're not good enough, to give up, to not try. That's the outsider. Much like the Stephen King's monster from his book *The Outsider,* it is good at blending in despite being a different creature than humans. It's a voice that sounds a lot like yours and is excellent at convincing you that you're not good enough. He's been around for thousands of years tormenting and tricking human beings into believing his dribble, but it's all a lie.

After spending months leading up to my surgery, getting berated by the outsider, it only amplified to insanity-inducing levels after my surgery. I couldn't go a minute without hearing him whispering quick but subtle jabs to my psyche.

*This is your life now, it isn't going to get better.*

*You're not strong enough for this, God is punishing you.*

*No one is coming to save you.*

That last one got me thinking, and it was partially true. I say "partially" because my family did everything in their power to save me, so the outsider wasn't accurate (like always), but that last line triggered a thought process that would save my life. After months of suffering, it became apparent that *no one can save me, but myself.*

Much like the saying "You can lead a horse to water but you can't make it drink," well, that was the reality of my life. My family and close friends were trying to get me to the water, practically dragging me to it, with it glistening right under my lips. None of that would mean squat if I didn't put my head down, cup my hands, and begin to drink.

My life was encompassed in pain for months, and I was aware of the suffering I was going through. The outsider convinced me the world should stop and give me sympathy, and anyone who didn't do that must have thought I wasn't important enough. What made me realize the outsider is precisely that, *an outsider,* and not myself, is when I saw the real pain I was causing to my family through my actions.

After that moment, I made the choice to not let my circumstances and the outsider write the rest of my life story. I was going to write it myself, and it sure as hell wasn't going to be a sad ending. It didn't happen with the flip of a switch, it took hard work and brutal honesty with myself. I had to address my insecurities head on and find a way to drown out the noise from the outsider. I had to be there for my family and learn to put on a mask to hide my pain to spare them from any suffering. I had to take responsibility for my health and to not let my condition dictate how I was going to live my life. I decided to be the author of my own truth and to take the pen back from the negative powers working against me.

If you are holding this book in your hands right now, odds are that you too have had bad encounters with the outsider. Perhaps you believe life is punishing you and there is no way out from your circumstances. I'm living proof there is a way out, and there is more to your life despite the hand you've been dealt.

I hope those facing adversities in their life can read my story and realize the power you have when it comes to controlling your attitude. The key thing to remember is that no one chooses to be ill with any medical condition. No one chooses the cards we've been dealt; life just gave them to us. It's up to us how we choose to play the hands we've been given. We are all responsible for the experiences that happen to us, even the ones we wished never did.

At the end of the day, we can either wallow in our circumstances, or we can live our lives courageously, compassionately, and honestly—courageous in the face of adversity, compassionately toward one another as we all suffer, and honestly so you live with no regrets and no shame. This way, others who are lost in similar circumstances can look up to someone who inspires them to change.

# PART I

# SPEED BUMPS
# & POTHOLES

# CHAPTER 1

# A NEW REALITY

———

Confusion was my main emotion as I sat there on the couch. My parents were explaining everything that was about to happen to me, but I couldn't grasp the severity of the words coming out of their mouth. I was zoned out in my own thoughts, blankly staring off into space as they were talking.

"Michael." My mother leaned forward to study my face. "Do you have any questions about what I just told you? I know I said a lot, it's normal to have questions."

I was like a character in a movie when the camera pans in on their face and the voices around them slowly fade out until we're looking right into their eyes. Then I snapped out of it and looked up at my mom, and her worried face looked back at me. She sat next to me on her favorite spot on the couch, the one she's sat on since we moved into our home when I was only two. Her red cup of tea was emitting a faint trail of steam as her hand gripped it to take a sip. Just behind her glasses, she wore an expression of guilt and fear in her eyes. My dad was sitting on the other side of me. He attempted to comfort me by patting my back in a circular motion. I gathered my thoughts and finally spoke.

"Yeah, I'm fine. I mean, you said everything is going to be okay, right?"

"You're going to be just fine, son. This is just a bump in the road. Remember that," my dad interjected, rubbing my back some more.

My mother looked at me with an expression that indicated she knew this wouldn't be the last time we would need to talk about what was happening. There would come a time where I would have a million questions.

"Okay, well, just know that if you need anything explained further. You can always ask me or your father. We've thrown a lot at you; it's normal to not understand something."

How could I truly understand what they had just told me and actually have a question? I was an eighteen-year-old kid in the middle of my senior year of high school at the time. A lot goes through the mind of a senior on a good day. What's my life going to be like after this year? What do I even want to do moving forward? At this point in my in young life I was having an identity crisis just dealing with normal everyday teenage stuff, lost in the moment, scattering to figure out who I wanted to be.

I was without a tribe, so to speak, and anything sounded better than nothing. I'd be on the Island of Misfit Toys if it meant having a feeling of camaraderie. Prior to my diagnosis, I was already feeling alienated among my peers, and that feeling was about to be amplified to Arthur Fleck levels. What I failed to realize at the time is that being a part of a group takes a degree of commitment, like being a part of a sports team or achieving academic excellence. They require sacrifice and hard work to earn those badges. I wanted to reap the rewards of these things without putting in an ounce of the work.

That's because I wasn't truly in tune with who I was at eighteen years old. I didn't bother to invest my time strengthening my hobbies, and truth be told, I didn't have many hobbies. I wasn't living, I was simply existing at this point. I was looking to plug a small leak in my life, when the uncomfortable truth was, I wasn't dealing with a small leak I was dealing with a complete decay in the foundation of who I was.

Throughout my life, I feel like there has been three different versions of myself; Mike in high school, Mike during recovery, and Mike after he has recovered. If you have ever watched *The Chappelle Show*, it's like the three Dave's skit. Mike in high school wanted all the rewards with none of the work. He would let his friends do his homework because he was too lazy and put a third of the effort into his assignments which would result in mediocre grades. He didn't participate in extracurricular activities; his after-school activity of choice was a three-hour nap. Mike in high school often took the easy way out and wondered why he wasn't feeling satisfied with himself. Reflecting back on him, it's hard to believe that was me at one point.

In the meantime, I was trying to enjoy my last year with the kids I grew up with. I wanted to focus on the typical fun high school stuff during your senior year—at least the things that are supposed to be fun, like hanging with friends around a bonfire on a crisp fall night with the added warmth of whatever cheap booze we could abscond from our parents' liquor cabinets. Or, going to the park on a warm hot sunny day, playing pick-up basketball, where tensions would bubble up underneath the surface until an unnecessary altercation would break out. It would usually be over a semi-competitive game with a bunch of immature teens who suffered from inflated egos.

I was too naive at the time to worry about anything outside of those things. What kid in high school could possibly understand the complexities of life?

What was I supposed to think or feel when my parents told me I was diagnosed with familial adenomatous polyposis? I wasn't a genius when it came to science or the human body; I didn't know what this condition was. I could barely pronounce the name of it at the time, and I was supposed to fully accept or understand it? That wasn't possible, not initially at least. It took some time for me to realize the severity of what they had told me.

This is the first time the outsider entered my life and began to taunt me. I was in denial of my situation and didn't want to accept what was happening to me. I thought if I pretended it wasn't real, that I could proceed with living carefree again. The reality was that it only made my situation worse, and the subtle jabs directed my way were only going to increase. The tension was beginning to bubble beneath the surface, sooner or later it was going to manifest itself into something much worse.

Eventually the outsider's presence could no longer be ignored. His voice had increased in decibels from a mere whisper to a normal talking tone that couldn't be shrugged off. I listened to him as he wasn't intimidating or even unreasonable. He resembled my subconscious internal dialogue, therefore I assumed it was myself trying to show me the light—especially since I had been running away from any shred of reality with my health situation. His words harbored some truth, which led me to believe his rhetoric. That was the bait, and he got me hook, line, and sinker. I began to buy into the narrative that this was going to be too much for me to handle. This symbiotic relationship we formed appeared honest at first but would soon turn volatile.

A couple of months prior to the news being shared with me, I got tested for the gene. It was a gorgeous Saturday morning when my mom woke me up. The beaming rays of sunshine peaked through my curtains and lit up slivers of my room with light. It wasn't the dog days of summer anymore, but it was a comfortable seventy-degree day, which was personally my favorite time of the year. The summertime can be a bit too hot for me, but today was perfect. A crisp enough breeze to stave off the occasional sweat beads, but never to the point where you felt chilly.

I remember my mom telling me the night before that I would have to get blood work done in the city the following morning. She didn't tell me what I was being tested for; she just said it wasn't a big deal and I had to get it done as a precaution. She told me that my older brother, Nicholas, had to get it done when he was my age so I figured it couldn't be that big of a deal since my brother was perfectly fine.

I dressed in shorts and a T-shirt, grabbed my Beats, and we got in the car and headed off toward the city. I wasn't really asking any questions as my parents' demeanor didn't make it seem like it was a big deal. My mind was preoccupied with the insignificant things that immature eighteen-year-old boys process on a daily basis. Like playing *Call of Duty* with my friends when I got back—you know, the important things in life.

I felt totally lost among my peers as most of the students I went to high school with appeared to have life all figured out at such a young age—at least that's what the outsider had convinced me of. My peers and friends had their sights set on becoming doctors, teachers, or going into the service.

They all had a plan set in motion at the beginning of their senior year. Some were getting full rides to colleges on athletic scholarships. Others were applying and getting accepted into their dream schools.

Little did I know at that age that nobody has it all figured out. If someone is telling you they have it figured out at eighteen, they're either lying or they have a God-given talent like no other that pretty much has them set in stone to be a success, like Lebron James being crowned "the chosen one" while he was still in high school. Or Justin Bieber becoming a teenage heartthrob because of his vocal talent, sprinkled in with his majestic mop that started a trend of teenage boys trying to capture the eyes of young girls by copying the bowl look. (Hey, I was one of them too. What can I say, the ladies loved the Biebs). Needless to say, I didn't have the same effect on the ladies as the Biebs did. Unless you had a situation like that presented in front of you, no eighteen year old has life figured out.

*\*\**

We arrived at Mount Sinai hospital to get my blood work done. No one told me what I was getting tested for. Even though I was beginning to question what was going on, I never would have imagined I was being tested for a rare genetic condition. I sat in the chair and waited until they called for me and then proceeded to feel the uncomfortable pinch as my blood was taken. It was quick and painless, and my mom and dad were by my side reassuring me as I went through it.

"Alright, Mr. Caprio, the results will be back in roughly two weeks or so. We will let your parents know when we get the results. Have a great weekend!" said a nice woman by the name of Karen.

That was it, a quick in-and-out appointment no longer than an hour. Part of me was thinking, *Couldn't we have just done this at our local doctor's office? What was so special about this place that they had to do it? Why were we in New York City to get blood work?* My questions were short lived, as I quickly forgot about them because my mom and my dad treated me to a day in the city.

This would become the typical protocol for our city trips to visit our surgeons. It would take roughly an hour to get to our destination, so it was a bit of an inconvenience to go to New York for doctor's appointments. Not to mention that driving in the city is a fever dream of people perpetually in a rush, blowing their horns at you for the most minuscule of driving errors, and if you're lucky enough you may get a couple of flattering four-letter words hurled your direction. On that particular day we ended up going to some restaurant on Madison Avenue that my dad thought looked appealing. Sometimes we would find ourselves at the Body Exhibit or the Intrepid. We turned into NYC tourists as a result of our doctor's appointments.

I remember sporadically throughout the six months between my blood work and receiving my diagnosis, I would ask my mom if the results came back. I remember the first time I asked her, it was roughly two weeks after my blood work. I was sitting down at the table in our dining room, eating dinner, and she was in the kitchen making herself a cup of tea, which is her usual routine every night around dinner time. I remember casually asking her, "Hey Mom, did we ever get those results back yet?"

"What results?" she asked with curiosity, as she was surprised that I remembered.

"You know, the blood work we got done. They said it would take two weeks. Have you heard anything yet?"

"Oh... No sweetie, something happened, and they got delayed. I'll let you know when I find out."

Looking back at it I should've taken that as a red flag. My mom was caught off guard and was surprised that I even remembered. She had bought herself some time, but she knew that she would have to tell me the results at some point. You see, what my mom was doing was protecting me from myself. She knows I tend to overthink situations, and she didn't want me to spend my entire senior year panicking and worrying; she wanted me to enjoy myself as best as I could. She was trying to protect me from the traumatizing experiences she went through when she had to endure the same thing.

When my mom was thirteen, she found out she had FAP. She spent the years leading up to her surgery feeling like a bit of an outcast. People would point at her signaling she was the one who had the condition amongst her sisters at the time. Not to mention how mentally taxing it was to marinate in the reality of having a rare condition as a child, knowing that eventually you're going to get cut open. At the time, I wasn't aware this condition was genetic and that my mom had it as well. All these years spending time and living with my mom, I never asked her any questions or even noticed anything out of the ordinary with her.

She debriefed me about a week later on the results of my blood test. Slowly and gradually over time, she told me everything I needed to know. Turns out she wasn't the only person in the family with FAP; my grandma and my Aunt Maria also had it. Throughout all these family vacations and all the time spent with one another, I never noticed a thing. My mom has a pretty big scar across her stomach, but I always assumed it was from pregnancy and never really thought too much of it. My aunt has the same scar I have, which is a relatively small scar compared to my mother's. My grandma had never worn a two piece, but I always assumed she just didn't like the style of that bathing suit. I never paid much attention to these subtle hints throughout the years. My mom explained to me what the condition was and explained the surgery to me, but they didn't tell me the full extent of the details right away.

I felt some of the stress and burden of knowing I held a deadly gene in the months that followed this life-altering news, but I'd say it has been something that's taken time over the years to sink in. Now that I'm an adult, I feel the cumbersome responsibility of my situation much more. Intimate relationships have an added level of personal responsibility on my shoulders knowing that if I have a child, I could be passing this condition onto another generation of my family. That is no easy burden to bear, and although at eighteen years old it didn't mean much, that would change in my twenties.

The last punch was thrown when I found out that for the rest of my life I'd have to undergo regular endoscopic checks to make sure the polyps don't spread in unwanted areas. I am at risk for a list of other cancers, such as small intestine, stomach, thyroid, pancreas, central nervous system, and bile ducts, all because of this stupid gene; although it should be noted these cancers affect less than 10 percent of affected individuals. It still isn't easy all the time, even to this day, to know all these very important bodily organs of mine have a slightly higher chance of failing me.

My mind was already cluttered with uncertainty, and it was about to get more doubts piled onto its tired self.

# CHAPTER 2

# MEET THE DOCTORS

———

In the coming months, I had three visits with my surgeon and his staff. The one thing my parents reassured me of was that our surgeon was the best there was. They described to me a brilliant, kind, and caring man by the name of Dr. Gorfine. They told me wonderful stories about him and how he was going to save and change my life. I believed their stories because they were all doing well. However, I also thought that maybe my parents were trying to overly reassure me, so I was anxious to judge this man when I met him for myself.

We were getting ready to see him for the first time in the spring of 2015. Even if he has the most gifted hands on the planet and a bunch of shiny plaques with his name written all over them, he's still a stranger to me. I was putting my health and my trust into someone I have never met before, and who was going to determine what the remainder of what my life would look like. That's a thought that can deeply trouble a grown man, let alone a teenager.

My mind was running laps, and I was ready to see him for myself. We got in the car and mentally prepared ourselves to drive through the twilight zone that is New York. If you couldn't tell by now, driving in the city is not fun. After we trudged through the sea of angry city dwellers with no scratches we walked over to his office.

In the waiting room, I was jittery, and I kept moving my legs; Dad and Mom noticed.

"Hey, it's going to be alright buddy. Just relax," my dad said as he put his hand on my shoulder.

After about fifteen minutes which felt like an eternity at that point, we were called in by a young-looking nurse. She brought us into the back room, and we passed four or five offices until we arrived at the last door on the right. I walked in and before I noticed him, I saw an impressive display of plaques and awards enshrining his office. His walls were covered with awards and articles of the "Top 100 Doctors in New York." Every square inch of his office was illuminated with plaques that celebrated his surgical brilliance.

Countless articles decorated him as one of the best surgeons in not only the city, but the country as well. He had gold commemorations from medical associations and organizations with big fancy names that I'd never heard of. I don't think there was room in his office for another award if he were to get another one. Quite literally, his success was looking me in the eyes, and it felt like his awards were pointing at me and laughing for even conceptualizing the slightest doubt in this man. With the amount of prestigious praise, I felt like I was about to meet a celebrity. Finally, I snapped out of being starstruck and made eye contact with Dr. Gorfine, who was sitting at his desk.

"Hello Michael, it's nice to finally meet you," he said with a comforting smile.

"I've heard a lot about you." I replied.

"Only good things, I hope?" He chuckled.

I sat down and took in his appearance for the first time. His short, white hair was a little messy. Just below his thick, bushy eyebrows, a pair of glasses rested on his nose. He was slightly taller than me but didn't tower over me. The aroma of a stale cigarette and coffee dominated the room. A sculpture of the very thing he was going to remove from me sat on his desk, right by his name plate.

My parents had described a person who seemed like a superhero, and his accolades made me feel like I was about to meet a larger-than-life figure, but in his office, I realized Dr. Gorfine was just a person too, like anyone else. He wasn't some divine spirit that can heal people with the snap of a finger. He was a human being with flaws, worries, and concerns just like the rest of us—except the work he did is something I could never do in a million years.

"So, I'm assuming you have a lot of questions. You are free to ask away, that is why we are here today," he said with his hands crossed at his desk, giving me his undivided attention.

I looked over at my mom, and she gave me a nod to encourage me. "It's okay, sweetie. Ask your questions. That's why we're here."

"Yes that's true. I don't get paid to look pretty," Dr. Gorfine said, easing the tension.

"Okay, well, is it going to feel any different when I have to go to the bathroom? Like when you have to go to the bathroom, you feel… the pressure, I guess is how I would describe it." I tried to figure out a smooth segue to this embarrassing, rambling mess of a question. "Being that I'm going to lose my large intestine is that going to… change? I'm sorry if that is a dumb question."

A weird question maybe, but I had a million weird questions. Let's face it, when you're losing your large intestine, there is bound to be some shit-related questions.

"Take a look around my office, I'm not the guy you should be embarrassed to ask shit-related questions to," he joked. My family and I got a nice chuckle out of that one. "But yes, it will be the same pressure-type feeling. That doesn't change at all."

"We will stay on the related topic then," I countered, before diving into my next question. "How many times will I be going to the bathroom in a day?"

"At the beginning, after the initial takedown surgery, it's going to be a lot. As time goes on, it will get better. By the time you have fully recovered, it usually ranges from two to six times a day, on an average day."

That answer stung a little bit to me. I wasn't really sure how to digest that news. I already began to feel the insecurities associated with my condition.

"Will I still be able to eat the foods I enjoy? Will I have to make changes to my diet?"

"Yes, you should be able to enjoy the same foods that you enjoy today. Maybe down the road, you'll have to make subtle diet changes, but that goes for anyone. Even I have to make diet changes with a normal system," he said reassuringly.

"Okay, that's a fair answer that I can live with." My turn to ask questions was over, and now it was time for Dr. Gorfine to tell me all the potential risks from the surgery.

He leaned forward in his chair. "Mom and Dad, I have to give him the full medical disclosure now."

"Oh." My mother frowned in disappointment. "Do you really have to do that? Can't I just sign off on it without him hearing this?" asked my mother frantically.

"Well, he is a legal adult at eighteen years old, I have to tell him."

My mom sat back looking unhappy and I wondered what he was about to tell me. "Alright sweetie, just remember he has to tell you this legally. Try not to freak out."

*Oh great, I can't wait to hear this.*

"Alright Michael, this is just the full medical disclosure. I'm going to tell you these scary things that rarely happen if ever. I have to say this legally in case one of them happens. If they happen and I don't warn you, my practice can get shut down."

He told me it was possible for me to go impotent for the rest of my life if a wrong nerve is struck, but then he said that only happens 1 percent of the time. He then said I could get blood clots in my legs that could lead to strokes and/or death. Death was one of the first things he warned me about.

After he told me *death*, I kind of spaced out into another world, my mind going a thousand miles a minute. I was only eighteen. I'm just starting my life. *How could it be possible that I could die? This couldn't be really happening to me. How could this be?*

I was in a panic as the room began to spin. I tried to look into his eyes and comprehend what he was saying. My heart rate increased dramatically, my palms started to sweat, and I felt like I was going to throw up. He was still telling me about the warnings, so I tried to focus.

"I know that is a lot to take in right now but trust me that these things rarely occur. I don't expect any of what I went over to happen. The only thing that has a realistic probability is that this surgery may need to be done in two parts, meaning you might need an ostomy." His reassurances made me feel a little better, but I was still a nervous wreck and my mind was running everywhere. He continued, "The surgery itself, whether it is two parts or one, will still happen like this. The large intestine needs to be removed completely, nothing left of it. That is where the polyps are, that's what's threatening your life. After we do that, we stretch the small intestine so that it covers up more space, so you aren't going to the bathroom as frequently," he said, pointing a pencil at a diagram of the human intestines. He was teaching us the procedure like we were students in his class. "Then I'm going to construct and make a J-pouch out of the end of the small intestine." He did a good job making something incredibly complicated sound routine. To him, though, it was routine; he has done thousands of these pouches.

A J-pouch is when they take the end of the small intestine, the ileum, and create a J-shaped pouch and hook it up to my anus to replace the job of the large intestine.[6] There really is no way to sugarcoat what it is. He was basically restructuring my intestines and my digestive system to work as normally as possible.

The thought of having to live with a bag was a nightmare situation for me, more so than the uncertainties with the J-pouch procedure. Having a hole in your abdomen, where your intestine is sutured into the skin on the outside, is not a very pleasant thought. I was also reassured that the odds of me having to have one was 20 percent. I tried to collect myself as if the odds were in my favor and I shouldn't have to worry about it. The meeting concluded, and we shook hands again before leaving the office.

---

6   Minesh Khatri, "Ulcerative Colitis Surgery: J-Pouch (IPAA) and Ileostomy Explained," WebMD, January 27, 2020.

My first experience with Dr. Gorfine showed him to be just as my parents described. As he was telling me the bad news, he was very calm, and I believed him when he told me it was going to be alright. I knew he wasn't lying to protect me. He let me know that because it was in his hands, he would not let me down. He's also legally obligated to not lie to me. That was my first of three meetings with him prior to the surgery. The second meeting was something that was a little more out of my comfort zone and made me feel like a "patient" for the first time.

## OUT OF MY ELEMENT

My second doctor's appointment was in New Jersey this time, not in the city. I was going to someone who works under Dr. Gorfine. His name was Dr. Morton, and what he did was colonoscopies and other scope tests. When my mom told me about this appointment, I felt an onslaught of different emotions.

For one, I was scared as hell. *A colonoscopy—isn't that what fifty-year-old men get? Why am I getting this?* Given the nature of my condition, I probably should have expected this to happen; but even then, you can't really prepare for the actual situation. How could I prepare myself mentally when I had to clear my intestines out so that a man in a white coat can insert a camera up my butt and examine my insides? Exactly, you can't prepare for something like that. Secondly, I was extremely embarrassed. It felt violating in many ways. Little did I know this was just the tip of the iceberg in regard to embarrassing things happening to me.

This was happening in the middle of the school year too. I was shell-shocked in all of my classes.

The outsider was now planting seeds in my mind all day with his toxic suggestions. He was reminding me, over and over again, about the hell that waits in front of me. I was already a slacker in high school with little to no motivation prior to this news. Now there was really no motivation to try and improve myself, I submitted defeat, which is precisely what the outsider's goal was. Teachers in my class wondered why I wasn't participating more. My friends wondered why I was even more distant. This is when anxiety entered my life.

Every morning that I woke up for school leading up to the colonoscopy, I faced a wave of anxiety. The first thing on my mind would be the bad news I was given. The outsider wouldn't let me sleep anymore, as our symbiotic relationship became more codependent. He would begin his nonsensical chirping at the crack of dawn in sync with the birds outside, and later into each night. Pretty soon I started to catch onto the outsider's tricks as I felt conflicted within myself. I couldn't be thinking about these things, right? Then I couldn't breathe; my chest was starting to tighten up. Met with that feeling was this overwhelming sense of doom, my mind would immediately race to figure out how to stop it.

The problem was I couldn't stop it, so this happened every single day. Much like I touched on in the introduction, my body was perceiving the bad news I had received as an existential threat: activating my sympathetic nervous system, which would pump adrenaline through my veins and energy to the outsider. It was out of my control at this point. He hijacked my mind, so I'd be living in a perpetual state of fear.

The bad thoughts and anxiety being inflicted on my life had no end in sight. No distraction could stop the outsider from persistently badgering me. At first, I would try to fight it and the bad thoughts that littered into my head from my shoulders. After a while, I began to marinate in these thoughts, and I started to become lethargic. Lying in bed trying to sleep at night would be disrupted by quick, painful thoughts that would act as an electric jolt to my awareness.

*What if you die?*

*You're not strong enough to handle this.*

*You might have an ostomy; you really think you can handle wearing a bag?*

*People are going to judge you for your condition. They're going to notice.*

Each one of those thoughts would pierce through my mind and make me wince in my bed as I tried to allow my brain to turn off. The outsider officially robbed me of my eight hours of sleep each night. I was now at his mercy. Whenever he took a rest, I was able to rest, which was never for long. He only seemed to need a handful of hours off at a time before he was fueled up for another day of bullying my subconscious. I was drained of my energy. Even if I wanted to fight back, I couldn't.

After a while, I just didn't care anymore. I became low energy; it was like they had sucked the energy out of me entirely, like a leech. I was now a shell of myself, as it appeared my parasitic relationship with the outsider had shifted to living rent free in my head, synonymous with my consciousness.

I didn't vent to anyone about these feelings because, personally, I thought I was losing my mind. When it feels like your own thoughts have been hijacked by some negative spirit, and turned against you, you would feel pretty crazy too. Imagine explaining that feeling to somebody. Now imagine trying to explain that to high schoolers. *Horrifying, I know.*

I got home from school the day before my colonoscopy, and my parents were home; they had taken the day off. When I got home it was preparation time, and this was a horrible experience. I had to drink a bottle containing this liquid that tasted like some industrial cleaner. It had a pure chemical taste to it, and the smell was so strong it shot up my nostrils and right to my brain. It was one of those smells that would give you a headache if you breathed it in too long—like cologne or gasoline, except I had to drink this vile liquid. I mixed it with Gatorade, but it didn't do much at all.

"Listen, I know it doesn't smell the best, but you have to drink it," pleaded my mother.

"I really have to drink all of that?" I glanced at the cocktail nauseously.

"The quicker you drink it, the closer you get to eating real food again."

Well damn, if there is a way to bribe me to drink a nasty laxative, it is to remind me I can eat again if I just go through with the process.

It took me a half hour to guzzle it down, and my stomach immediately started to rumble. Within minutes, the preparation began to do its job as I ran back and forth to the bathroom for the remainder of the night. After going to the bathroom all night, it finally ended, and I was as empty as I could get. Now it was time to wait for my appointment in the morning.

## COLONOSCOPY

We arrived at the doctor's office bright and early, and we waited for them to call my name. I began to get antsy, as I was surrounded by a bunch of older people going for their routine colonoscopies, and then there was me, basically a kid.

I could only imagine why these people thought I was going to be getting a scope at such a young age.

"Michael Caprio," the nurse called for me, as it was my time. I nervously shuffled past the other patients as they waited to get violated. She slapped a wristband on me, and I was guided into the back room.

The new area I was brought to was like a mini hospital. There were five or six little beds with curtains for privacy by them and the room they would wheel you into. They first made me sign off on this legal paper letting me know the risks of everything I was going through. They told me to sign at the bottom just above my name. Something caught my eye. The paper said I acknowledged there is a possibility I could die or slip off into a coma and the hospital wouldn't be held responsible or something to that effect.

I stopped and stared at it, and my mind began racing. The issue for me wasn't what was going to happen that day, but it made me realize the severity of everything I was going to go through. In the future, I would have to sign the same exact piece of paper for both of my operations, and I realized then that this was life or death for me. It was something I would have never imagined. It never became easier down the road either; I just accepted the reality better. Reading those words on that piece of paper will always be sobering and surreal.

"So, Michael, I'm going to assume this is new to you," Dr. Morton said jokingly.

I cracked a slight smile through my nerves, even though I terrified.

"This is going to be easy I promise you. You're going to be hooked up to the IV, and we are going to count back from ten. By the time we reach one, you will be asleep and then when you wake up you will be all done. No pain, I promise. Easy as pie," he said reassuringly.

After the rundown, they hooked me up to an IV and told me to count down from ten. At around three, my eyes forced shut, it felt like a weight was pulling down on them. Then after my eyelids flapped shut, darkness ensued.

For a colonoscopy, the doctor waits until you're asleep, and once you are, he inserts a colonoscope in your rectum to observe what is going on inside your colon. The colonoscope looks like a three-eyed snake. On the tip of the colonoscope is a camera so that the doctor can receive real time images of your colon as he maneuvers his way around. The other two eyes on the snake are a light, as you can imagine—not much sun shines down there. The last remaining eye of the snake is a tool used to deploy air or water into the colon. The water is to clean out any waste blocking the camera. The air is used to expand your colon so nothing is hiding in any nooks and crannies.

Then the last utensil on the colonoscope is where the surgical tools propel themselves out from, which looks like the second mouth from Ridley Scott's *Alien*. The surgical tools propel themselves out when a polyp is spotted, and the tool is used to extract the polyp for a biopsy to see if the tissue from which the polyp grew is cancerous. In my case, they were only observing to see if the polyps were there, none were removed.

I woke up a little high from the anesthetics. The nurses came in and were giving me instructions. During the instructions, I faded out of reality and into my own thoughts. Though in the long run, this whole experience was really a cake walk compared to what I would go through in the coming months; but it did make me feel like a patient. That was something I didn't like to admit to myself. I never wanted to accept any of this during the entire process. I wanted to look at myself as a person who was normal. I wasn't ready to let go of that sentiment.

The reality was that this wasn't normal, and I knew of no one outside of my family going through something like this—none of my friends or the people I went to school with or worked with. No one. I felt like an outcast that had no outlet to vent my emotions too. Who could understand what I was going through?

At the time, I was too scared and embarrassed to talk to my family members who had the gene about what I was going through. I guess talking to my family about it would make it a reality. I guess part of me was trying to ignore the people I did have to talk to about it. I was scared, depressed, confused, and had a bunch of morbid thoughts going through my head. I didn't know if telling them all these things would scare them or make me look weak for thinking these things—which is entirely foolish in hindsight. As time would go on, the bond between me, my grandma, my aunt, and my mother would strengthen through our experience of having one of the rarest conditions on this planet.

The results for my colonoscopy were shown to me before we left the facility that day. As I was looking at these pictures, the reality set in that I really had this condition.

"Well, as we basically expected, the results show that the blood tests were accurate," explained Dr. Morton as he showed me the pictures inside my colon. "Those little bumps are the polyps, and as you can see, there are quite a few of them. I would operate as soon as possible—the younger, the better."

My intestines were lined with an innumerable amount of these little polyps. It was like my intestines were lined with bubble wrap; it was truly mind-blowing what I was looking at. I was only eighteen, I was healthy, I had nothing wrong with me at the time; and yet inside of me, these polyps were just growing—growing and multiplying at an alarming rate, all out of my sight.

I had a solution for me fortunately, and that solution was the surgical brilliance of Dr. Gorfine. In just a few short months, those polyps that were slowly invading my large intestine would be no more. There would be no more large intestine, period. I was fortunate enough to be tested at a young age, so the silent and deadly polyps had no chance for the surprise attack they had planned on me.

# CHAPTER 3

# BAD HABITS

———

When I got home, I started a habit that would only worsen over the next couple of months before my surgery. It is a bad routine everyone tells you not to do: I Googled my condition on the internet. I read horror story after horror story of what my condition did to people. I was reading about those who had desmoid tumors and other complications from this disease, stuff I was never told about. My trust in everything being told to me evaporated with each article I read. *Why wasn't I being told these things?*

On these forums regarding my condition I came across something so bizarre I couldn't believe it. Some patients reported having symptoms that had nothing to do with the digestive system. People with FAP develop bumps or lumps on their skull, jaw, legs, and arms. These benign growths are called desmoid tumors.[7] This oddly enough happened to me after my surgeries, when I developed a small bump on my head. People reported having cysts on the skin, and adolescents have issues with their baby teeth coming out.

———

7    "Familial Adenomatous Polyposis: MedlinePlus Genetics," MedlinePlus. US National Library of Medicine, August 18, 2020.

Teeth don't erupt from the jaw when they should. When I read those words, it resonated with me. It had been obvious I've had this condition since I was a child, when I had major dental issues.

During my early childhood, I had trouble with my baby teeth. They wouldn't fall out of my mouth, and my adult teeth would grow behind them. It was as if I had two rows of teeth, similar to a shark. When I was a kid, I had to get eighteen of my baby teeth pulled in one sitting. I have faint memories of my friends murmuring to me about how their teeth grew in easily and had to get one or two removed, max. Everyone was astonished I had to get so many teeth pulled in general, let alone all at once. Somehow, I still thought my situation was normal for most of my life.

My dental issues didn't end there, unfortunately. I had developed what is called a compound odontoma, which resembles a small collection of teeth that form in the jaw during tooth development.[8] Mine developed on the lower right side of my mouth right by my canine tooth. I had to go to an oral surgeon, who was fascinated I had it. This is the main reason I can still remember the name of the growth today from childhood. He had to cut my gum open and vacuum out all these little teeth fragments. He showed me the pile of bone fragments in my gums after the surgery, and all I could think was how the hell did all of that fit in my mouth? Since bone spurs and growths are common with my condition, my family and I now realize this was probably the best early warning sign I had the condition.

---

8    R Gedik, and S Müftüoğlu, "Compound Odontoma: Differential Diagnosis and Review of the Literature," *West Indian Medical Journal*, August 20, 2015.

As I got more curious and looked up my surgery, specifically the J-pouch, I saw more horror stories of people who went through the procedure and wished they had never done it. They discussed how their quality of life went down and how they couldn't eat normal foods or do everyday life activities. They wrote how they suffered from pouchitis, and this confused me. Does this surgery come with its own illness? I was reading about how pouchitis is a complication of J-pouch surgery, resulting in inflammation that occurs in the lining of the pouch.[9] At the time of this writing, I've had one bad bout of pouchitis, and it feels like a stomach bug on steroids. Reading those forums online couldn't prepare me for the first time I had pouchitis.

It happened when I worked at a liquor store two years after my initial surgeries. I had made a full recovery, while becoming acclimated with my new plumbing. Those articles I read on pouchitis had slipped my mind, and it was a normal night on the job. I was working with a co-worker who luckily was a friend, which made this night a bit less embarrassing. I was stocking the cooler and when I came out of the frosty room, my joints began to get sore. It felt as if I was beginning to get a fever. Next came the fatigue, and eventually my stomach began grumbling. After a couple minutes, I could tell something wasn't right, but I couldn't figure out what it was. The upset stomach turned into shooting dagger like pains throughout my abdomen. From there on, I spent the rest of the night limping back and forth from the bathroom holding my abdomen, begging for relief with none in sight.

---

9    "Pouchitis," Mayo Clinic, Mayo Foundation for Medical Education and Research, September 29, 2020.

I wasn't going to the bathroom; it wasn't like I had a case of the runs. It was the worst pain I had experienced since my initial surgery; I was begging to go at this point. I began to panic. *Am I having a blockage? Do I need to call 911?* It got to the point where I had to consider it not knowing what the hell was going on, and my co-worker shifted from busting my chops to genuine concern. He could see this wasn't just a stomach bug, and I had to come clean with him about my condition considering no one on the job knew at the time.

Luckily, he was a friend, as I mentioned before, and he understood by my body language I was not okay. So, I left and drove home, viscerally gripping the stirring wheel with each passing spasm. At first, the gut-wrenching spasms would happen for about five to ten seconds every minute. They started to get longer and happen more frequently. When I got home, I was in my bed under blankets shivering while wincing as my mother looked at me in horror. It wasn't until she called my aunt, who has had a couple of bouts with pouchitis when we were able to diagnosis it. She immediately recognized the symptoms, so we called Dr. Gorfine for help. He prescribed a medication over the phone, and told me it would clear things up, but I'd have to take it easy for a couple of days.

The medicine helped within the first six hours, and I finally began to feel human again. The whole situation was scary, but luckily the solution can be easily applied once it's recognized. What my experience with pouchitis made me realize, which I lacked in the moment when I was eighteen, was that this complication effects FAP patients far less than it does anyone with an inflammatory bowel disease like Crohn's or Colitis. Their intestines get inflamed on a far more regular basis, and I can't say I blame those people for expressing their grievances online. If I lived in the pain and

I experienced that night on a daily basis, I'd go mad. It just goes to show you this option isn't as ideal for other people as it was for me.

Reading all of this was too much, and I was devastated. My mind was racing a million miles a minute. I was so overwhelmed I thought I was going to throw up and pass out. The prospect of what my life could look like after surgery terrified me. The last thing I wanted was to end up like one of these people I was reading about.

All of a sudden, my views on things started to shift. In the beginning of this whole fiasco, I struggled immensely with exploring the idea of my mortality. Now, after reading about the people who lived through my surgery, imagining living their miserable existence after the fact was a 12-6 curveball I never anticipated. I didn't think it was possible for something to deter me from my fear of death at the time. It was a whole new dynamic added to the equation. We jumped straight from times tables to long division. Suddenly, I stopped worrying about dying so much, and my focus shifted to the possibility my life wouldn't be worth living after the surgery.

These conflicting thoughts consumed all of my energy. I spent one day wrestling with the idea of death and the next marinating about potential despair after enduring the agonizing surgeries in front of me. One thing that was certain was my operation was going to be brutal and life changing. Imagine if I endure all that suffering, only to be perpetually miserable for the rest of my life. That sounded like a fate worse than death.

My thoughts were working overtime for the next couple of weeks. You know that *SpongeBob* episode where he loses his identity and he can't remember his name? Yes, I'm using a *SpongeBob* episode for a reference—deal with it. They show a visual representation of his thoughts, and it's a bunch of SpongeBobs running around his head shouting, while fire and chaos unravels. That was more or less how it felt inside of my mind for the coming weeks. I was constantly thinking about one of the two dilemmas I had.

I withdrew once again from socializing with my family and friends after reading these forums. Behaving in this strange manner for some time, my mother's instincts detected trouble.

"Michael, I need you to be honest with me," she said with concern in her voice.

"Yeah, what's up?" I asked, anticipating the question.

"Have you been researching your condition on the internet? I know you, and I can tell something's off. What have you been reading online?" she probed.

I cocked my head up at her as I was caught off guard that she knew what I was reading. "I've been reading about how this is more serious than you told me. People who have what I have write about how sad they are, how their lives are not good, and they're miserable. Is that really going to be me?"

She shook her head in disappointment. "You have to stay offline. When you meet with Dr. Gorfine this week you will realize there is absolutely nothing to worry about. It is normal to be scared and have questions. Address your questions with him. I promise you he will answer them all."

*Fair enough*, I thought to myself. I have to give the man a chance to answer my questions before I completely write him off as untrustworthy. I was just hoping he would give me the reassurance I so desperately needed.

When we finally had our final meeting with Dr. Gorfine, my mother was right. He debunked everything and I realized I was pretty naive. My condition is so rare the vast majority of people with J-pouches have a different illness then me. Most people who get J-pouches are people who suffer from ulcerative colitis or Crohn's disease. Both of these diseases are chronic diseases that have no known "cures." Treatment varies from patient to patient, and so does the severity of the disease. People with one of these conditions usually get the J-pouch as a last resort.

The main difference between those patients and myself was that my condition isn't chronic, and it doesn't affect the rest of my digestive system the way those conditions do. Dr. Gorfine explained to me that ulcerative colitis only involves the large bowel (colon and rectum) like my condition, but the flare ups that UC is known for don't occur with my condition. Crohn's disease can involve the entire digestive tract, anywhere from mouth to anus. A J-pouch is not generally performed on a patient with known Crohn's disease. That said, a number (around 10 percent) of patients thought to have UC at the time of J-pouch surgery later are thought to have had Crohn's disease all along. This change in diagnosis usually happens when a late complication develops after surgery. These complications don't happen with my condition.

My other fear from the blog posts online was pouchitis. I wanted to know what this was.

"So, what exactly is pouchitis? Is it something serious that I should be concerned about?" I asked.

"Pouchitis is something that doesn't happen often in my patients. It does happen though, and when it does happen, it has similar qualities to the common stomach bug. There will be some issues going to the bathroom, maybe a slight fever," he explained.

"Well, how long does it last? What do I do if I get it?" I questioned him further.

"Just call me, and I'll call in a prescription for this medicine that will eliminate it in a week. It'll last for three to five days. Then it will go away. Nothing more than that," he reassured me.

He was a man of his word.

The whole conversation I had with him that day took some major worries off my mind. I had begun to form my doubts with my surgeon prior to this meeting. From my perspective it seemed he tried to hide some valuable details from me. After his explanation, it made sense why it wasn't brought up in the initial meeting. I was already experiencing sensory overload. My doubts about Dr. Gorfine were really a product of my anxiety and my obsessive research online.

I was still nervous beyond words and couldn't shake the thoughts of the coming months, and more specifically, the date of my surgery.

After the conversation was over, we made it official. He got the paperwork, and we made the appointment at his office. I was looking at it on a piece of paper. I stared at it as my mom and the nurses were talking and making arrangements. There it was in ink: July 10, 10 a.m., Patient: Michael Caprio.

# CHAPTER 4

# NO TURNING BACK

---

I carried on the rest of my senior year trying to avoid thinking about the inevitable. I wanted to enjoy the last couple of months I had left before my body would become a marvel of medical engineering. July 11 felt like the last day of my existence as I knew it. Not only was I clueless on how I would deal with the challenges of the surgery and recovery that lay before me, but I also knew there could be a chance I wouldn't wake up at all. It was a sobering thought.

For the rest of the year, I lived my life as if nothing would be the same again. I stopped keeping track of my physique and ate whatever I wanted because I figured I should fatten up before I became a skeleton. Maybe it would off-set looking like a walking corpse. For the record, my hypothesis didn't hold up.

I engaged in a fair amount of drinking with my friends because when you're devoid of emotional maturity as a teenager, nothing is more attractive than a magical liquid that puts a chokehold on your subconscious thoughts—especially when you haven't the slightest clue on how to stop being so anxious. Also, when you grow up in a small suburban town there isn't a lot to do, which makes it an even more attractive combination. In hindsight, when I reflect on my behavior during this time, I realize now that I was running from my problems. I didn't have the ability to deal with emotional trauma back then. I was going through a Herculean life experience with no life tools under my belt yet. I had to learn in real time how to deal with it all. I didn't want to talk about what I was going through because talking about it made it real.

On weekend nights, I couldn't stay inside, so I'd do anything to get out of the house. Sitting in my room and basking in my nightmare scenarios was excruciating. I couldn't handle it. The outsider was winning this time and winning big. The thoughts that he inserted into my consciousness were overwhelming. It felt as if another thought were crammed into my crowded mind, that they would begin seeping out of my ears and stretching my cranium until it popped. *Where is the off switch?*

There were nights where nothing was going on in town—no party, no hangouts, no new movies I could watch, *nothing*. I was so determined to distract myself that sometimes I would pick a friend or two up and aimlessly drive for the night. Again, there isn't much to do in the dead of winter in good ole Hopatcong, so distractions were limited. Sometimes you had to get creative. Although driving around listening to music isn't exactly a groundbreaking idea, it did soothe the tension.

Time went by, and the surgery got closer. I went through milestones that should have excited me, like graduating high school and preparing for the next phase of my life. These are happy times for most normal high schoolers, but they weren't for me. My peers were celebrating and getting ready to spend our last summer together before we all departed, and I was preparing to have my whole life turned upside down and inside out.

There were no goodbyes or memories from my summer that year. I was able to enjoy the first week of July before I was hospitalized, which wasn't enough time to see many of the friends I had known all my life before they left for college or whatever was next for them. I still haven't seen some of those people to this day in fact. I had to postpone my plans to enroll in school; spring 2016 would be the earliest I'd be sitting behind a school desk again. This would be the best-case scenario.

The night before my surgery was surreal; no more time was left to blow off. There was no text message I could send to friends in a last-ditch effort to get out of the house for the night and escape. When I woke up, it would officially be the day I had been dreading for six months, but first, I had to take the same preparation I had before my colonoscopy. I also had to shower and apply a strong cleaner on my abdomen where I was going to be operated on. It became more and more real as each minute of my last night of being *me* slipped away.

I spent the remainder of the night with my family watching *The Sopranos*. Enjoying TV shows is a popular way of passing time in my household. It was also a way to bring the family together, and in a time like this, being together is what I needed. Also, what is more stereotypical than an Italian family binge-watching a show about Italian mobsters in New Jersey? We all needed it, and we all needed some normalcy to take our minds off of the realities of the next morning. Nothing helps you forget about a major surgery looming the next day than watching Tony Soprano verbally and physically assault people.

After we finished and it was time for some sleep, I lay in my bed staring off into space. *Bzzz. Bzzz.* Suddenly, my phone started to go off. I looked down to see text messages from my friends. People I told months ago who remembered tomorrow was the date I was going under the knife.

*Good luck tomorrow, buddy. Everything's gonna be alright.*

*I just remembered that tomorrow is the big day for you, I'm going to keep you in my prayers. Please text me when you wake up.*

*Keeping you in my thoughts, Michael. I know you're nervous—that's normal. You'll get over this.*

The wishes of good luck from my friends made me feel less alone in this fight. It also, however, made me a little scared of the severity of things. Some of my friends were also concerned as to what was going to happen. They remained positive that things would be okay, but small quirks in their messages and conversations with me prior to the surgery showed me they were anxious too.

As I lay down in my bed, I remembered what my dad had been saying throughout this entire time: "It's just a bump in the road." My dad had a very calm demeanor over the past six months. Yes, he was nervous and he showed it, but he was confident in the process. I put all the thoughts racing through my head that night to ease and just kept saying to myself, "It's just a bump in the road." I kept saying those words until my eyes got heavy, and I slowly shut my eyelids, welcoming sleep by accepting tomorrow was going to happen no matter how much I thought about it.

## TIME'S UP

It was early in the morning when my parents woke me up to get us prepared. We all hopped into the car at around 7 a.m. It was an ungodly time for me to be up that early, but for some reason, I wasn't bothered. I was ready to go and get this over with. I was met with a wave of anxious energy when I woke up which was the equivalent to C4 pre-workout. Not to mention, I was completely empty and hadn't had a meal in twenty-four hours. I was so hungry and ready to just eat. Little did I know my appetite would be non-existent for about eleven days after the surgery.

We got in the car and headed for Manhattan. I sat in the back seat with my Beats on zoning out of reality and into my music.

When we arrived at the hospital and parked our car in the parking garage across the street, it was an eerie sight. It was dead in Manhattan that morning as we walked into the hospital. Nothing was going on; we were the only people on the street at the time. The city that supposedly never sleeps seemed to be in a deep slumber. It was a beautiful summer morning with the sun illuminating behind the skyscrapers, and the pink glow of the sun made the sky and city look like something out of a postcard.

We walked in and familiarized ourselves with the check-in procedures. I was never aware of how much of a process it was to get operated on. First, we had to shuffle over to the general admission desk and recite the who, what, and why of my surgery.

"What's your name sir?" asked a hospital worker.

"Michael Caprio," I said in an anxious voice.

I observed my surroundings like a scared animal, watching nurses and doctors pass by me in their scrubs with cups of coffee in hand. I heard murmurs about operations and scheduling from bypassing conversations.

"Okay, and what is the operation you're having today, along with your surgeon?" he asked, trying to get my attention.

I looked over at my parents for approval, and they nudged me on to say it.

"I'm getting a J-pouch operation, I guess is what it's called, and my surgeon is Dr. Gorfine."

"Okay, just have a seat, and we'll call you into the next room when we're ready."

I waited in the first lobby for about ten minutes and was then brought into a second waiting area. This is when things got even more surreal. They put a patient bracelet on my wrist that had all the information I've been reciting back to the nurses and hospital workers. I sat nervously in the green padded chair, picking my cuticles as I read the words on my bracelet.

*Patient: Michael Caprio, Surgeon: Dr. Gorfine*

I zoned out slowly feeling the consuming grasp of the outsider when a nurse got my attention. It was time to go into the pre-operation room. I put on a hospital gown, placed all of my belongings into a bag, and then sat as I waited for my name to be called. My stomach was in knots, and I felt like I was going to vomit everywhere. I was shivering uncontrollably as if I was suffering from hypothermia. My parents were still by my side, and I tried to put on a strong face and hide my nerves. It didn't work.

"It's okay to be a nervous, sweetie. You're going to be fine. You're in the best hands with Dr. Gorfine," my mom said patting me on my back, trying to calm me down.

"Yeah, look at your mother. If she can do it, you can," my dad said jokingly, poking fun at my mom.

Then finally, two nurses came down and called my name, and we were taken into the elevator.

"No family members are allowed past this point, I'm sorry," the nurse said to my parents.

I began to panic, my heart racing. I looked at my mom almost to give her a signal to come with me.

"Excuse me, but he's still a kid. I don't care if he's a legal adult. This is very nerve-racking for him. Can we please stay with him? He needs us right now," my mom said with some attitude toward the nurse.

"Okay, that's fine then. You can stay with him. I'm sorry I didn't realize." The nurse was a little taken back by what my mom said.

I was fine with it; my mom knew I needed my family now more than ever.

We took the elevator up another some odd floors, and we arrived at the final step before the operating room. This is where I was set into the bed, and they hooked me up with IVs. I was in a room with about twenty other people who were waiting for their operations as well. There was one woman who was reading a book all calm and normal before her operation. I thought to myself, *How the hell is this woman so calm and relaxed before surgery that she can read a book?* I figured maybe it was a minor operation, but I still couldn't believe how she didn't seem nervous in the slightest bit.

The atmosphere became increasingly more disturbing as there was a man screaming and moaning prior to his surgery. I'm not sure if he had a condition, or had an issue where he was in a lot of pain, or just couldn't control his emotions. Regardless of what was causing him to moan and scream, it made the atmosphere in the room extremely unsettling and quite eerie. The last place you want to hear moans of displeasure and pain is a pre-operating room, as you try patiently to wait for your turn.

I was shaking in the bed and my parents noticed. "Can you please give him something to relax a little bit?" my mom whispered to the nurse who came in to check on me.

I'm not sure what it was that they gave me, but *man was it good*. I was starting to relax more and think less, as I began to accept my fate whatever it might be.

In came Dr. Gorfine after about five to ten minutes of talking with his assistant. He was in his scrubs this time, which made this whole situation a little more real to me than the previous times I had met with him.

"Remember Michael, you know what the most important part of all this is right?" he asked half-jokingly.

"Yes, to make you look good," I said cracking a smile.

Dr. Gorfine began talking with my parents after that, while the nurses got me ready to move. The reality was starting to set in more and more. It was about to happen. I couldn't even focus on what he was saying to my parents. I was just spacing out; words were no longer discernible. My mom then hugged Dr. Gorfine, and my dad shook his hand.

It was official. Dr. Gorfine was telling me to say my final goodbyes to my family.

My mom held my hand as my dad stood by her side rubbing her shoulders. "It's going to be okay. Dr. Gorfine is going to help you," she said and then proceeded to kiss my hand.

I looked up at them, uncertainty racing through my mind. I didn't know what to say; I was truthfully speechless.

"I hope so," I then mumbled quietly.

"I know so," my mom quickly answered. My dad looked on nodding his head. Words can't really do much in a situation like this. I think all of us understood that and kept our collective doubts internalized knowing that expressing them will only make the situation more unnerving.

We held a silent moment where we embraced before the inevitable ripped us away from each other. Dr. Gorfine came over to break up the family reunion.

"I know this part is always tough, but it's time to say goodbye," he said, standing by us waiting for our moment to be over.

"Goodbye, sweetie. We love you, and we'll be here when you wake up," my mom said as she stepped away to let Dr. Gorfine do his thing.

"You're going to be just fine, son. We love you," my dad added before Dr. Gorfine whisked me away. I watched their sad faces wave goodbye to me as they were in every parent's nightmare scenario. A scenario where they can no longer help, and they would just have to put the fate of their child in some else's hands.

As we were going down the hallway, there were operating rooms on the left and right. Doctors were popping in and out of these doors with bloody aprons on and some people were getting wheeled in just like I was. Seeing the blood on the aprons increased my heart rate, and I began to sweat. It was silent for the first moments as we were heading down but Dr. Gorfine broke the silence and cracked a joke with me.

"A lot of traffic here this morning, more so than usual," he said referring to the other patients getting wheeled up and down the hall. "I know this is scary and new to you. I promise you're going to be okay." There was no follow up joke this time from Dr. Gorfine; he meant business. He wasn't going to let me down.

We finally busted through the doors of the operating room, and I took it in. It was nothing like I imagined it to be. It was a relatively small room with an innumerable amount of medical equipment, and I didn't know what any of it was.

It threw me off thinking that all of this stuff was going to be used on me. The next thing I knew, I was being strapped onto an ice-cold operating table in a metallic room that bounced the light off every corner of my four-dimensional hell.

# PART II

# ROADWORK

## CHAPTER 5

# THE NEW NORMAL

———

I opened my eyes, and all I could see were the silhouettes of two faces in front of me. Behind them was a bright beaming white light. I couldn't see any details of the faces. It was just the outlines, parallel twin shadows with this holy light just beaming down in the backdrop.

I was foggy and felt light; I didn't feel real. It didn't feel like I was laying on anything. I couldn't sense my body or anything at all. I remember thinking to myself, *Am I dead? Is this what heaven is or is supposed to look like?* A couple seconds later they were talking to me and I realized it was my doctors asking me questions to confirm if I was conscious and functioning. I didn't know what they were asking me, and I wasn't sure if I was answering them properly. The whole thing to this day is extremely foggy and the only detail I remember asking them was, "Do...do I have..." It was a struggle to speak in the softest of tones. "...the bag?"

The two silhouettes looked at each other before the one on the right began to answer my question.

"Yes, yes you do," said the shadowy figure on the right who I assumed was Dr. Gorfine.

After that, it was back to darkness.

The next thing I remember was waking up in the post-op room. The room held a bunch of patients fresh out of surgery laying in their hospital beds with curtains on both sides for privacy. There was one nurse patrolling the room to make sure everyone was okay. Most of the patients were asleep, but I was forced awake from the terrible pain I was in. The pain was something I wouldn't wish on my worst enemy.

My abdomen felt comparable to being stabbed over and over again. It was a deep, stinging pain that was agonizing. I was laying on my back and I tried moving my arms and my legs, but I couldn't. My limbs felt like they weighed ten tons each. It took every fiber of my being to try and move them, but my body couldn't.

I remembered being told that when I woke up from my surgery, I would have a pain pump. So, I pieced this together as I was in a frantic battle to combat the pain, and I managed to muster up the strength to move my hand to see if I could find it. I was fumbling around by my waist searching for it and all of a sudden, I felt a little ball of something. It felt plausible that it could be a pump, so I started to squeeze it. Nothing was happening, so I turned my head to the right to examine the situation and was shocked at what I saw.

It was a little see-through plastic sack that had a blood-like fluid in it. It wasn't blood red but had more of a rose look to it. The sack was connected to a tube and I pulled on it to realize this thing was inside of my body. I pulled and felt a shooting pain go through my body and I groaned. Groaning hurt—any movement hurt. I was panicking, I couldn't find my pain pump, and not only could I not find it, but I also found these two drains that were connected to my hip.

I would later learn that those little sacks that were embedded in my hull are called Jackson-Pratt drains. Jackson-Pratt

drains are used to drain bodily fluids from surgery sites.[10]
Yes, for those of you wondering, it is just as painful as it
sounds.

I saw the nurse walking and I tried to get her attention.
Speaking was a near impossible task as trying to talk pulled
on my abdomen area and caused all sorts of pain. This experience would educate me on how everything we do is connected to our core area. It took me all the might in my body
to whisper the words, "Nurse...help...please."

By the grace of God, the nurse heard me and came over.
I was able to mouth the words pain pump, and she pieced
two and two together and tried to figure it out as to why I
didn't have one.

My missing pain pump would be an issue for the first
twenty-four hours post-surgery. The insurance company was
having an issue and for some reason, I couldn't get this pain
pump until the next morning. I had to go through the whole
first night with inadequate pain relief.

I nodded on and off for most of my stay in the post-op
room. I only remember waking up periodically to talk to my
family quick as they were checking on me to see how I was.

I then remember waking up as they were ready to wheel
me up to my room. I remember this experience because it
was traumatizing to me. They had to lift me up and put me
onto another hospital bed. When they grabbed my body, the
pain was so intense it threw my body into a spasm. My whole
body just started to twitch and shake randomly for ten to
fifteen seconds, each time more painful than the last. With

---

10    "Caring for Your Jackson-Pratt Drain," Memorial Sloan Kettering Cancer
      Center, Accessed January 9, 2021.

every crack we hit as they wheeled me up to my room it sent my body into a spasm attack.

These spasms were the worst part of the recovery process in the hospital. As we got settled into my room that night I was told to try and sleep. I couldn't though; every time I was about to, I was thrown into one of these unprovoked spasm nightmares. They were so painful, and I was so frustrated I started to cry. I was broken down; the pain was too much, and there was no solution in the near future. Father Time was going to be the only real solution to my pain, which is something I didn't want to accept.

My mom was quite frustrated with the nurses for not having the full arsenal of pain meds at my disposal. She was fighting with nurses to try and get me properly set up. Mom's persistence paid off after a couple of hours, when I was finally set up in the late hours of the night with the proper meds. Even after I got set up, my mom still was expressing emotions of guilt, which partially confused me at first but would make sense to me later on.

Part of the reason was that my mom felt guilty this was happening to me. This was her condition, her bad genes, and her choice to have kids knowing this was a possibility. This was eating my mom alive, and she couldn't leave me by myself. She made sure no one was going to come in and pick at my wounds who wasn't from Gorfine's medical team. She made sure I was going to get my pain meds. She was my protector.

She knew how scary it was to be in this spot by yourself because she lived through it. Back when she got her surgery, you had to be alone. My mom's experience in the hospital was not a good one, and she made sure that mine was the best it could possibly be. She made sure I was not alone, and for that,

I am forever thankful she stood by my side during my stay in the hospital because without her being there overnight, I'm not sure if I could've done it on my own.

## THE BATTLE BEGINS

My first trip in the hospital consisted of the longest eleven days of my life. It was almost like it was divided into two trips. The first couple of days were a blur; it seemed like they never happened. The memories I have I can't piece together to which day they belonged to.

I had to try and fill in the gaps only going off the information I was able to process those first couple days. So, it's hard to dig back to how I was feeling in those moments. They feel akin to a dream, not real or tangible. Long distant memories, that were so painful it's almost like my mind had to block out some of the details for my own protection. A defense mechanism to protect me from the horrifying realities hanging in the balance.

The medication I was prescribed was strong, and I was using my fair share to help deal with the pain, which is totally understandable when you're fresh off a nine-hour operation. The medication had a profound ability to put my emotional havoc into submission. The relentless barrage of self-pity and depression that was putting a devastating choke hold on my brain had met its match in the form of my IV, which was loaded with Percocet. With each press of a button, I administered a dosage that moved into my bloodstream. As they traveled throughout my body, the ongoing train wreck of emotions that we're chastising my conscious self were suddenly sedated and put to rest, along with my agonizing physical pain.

The severity of what was going on had taken a temporary back seat. I wasn't able to mentally grasp what was going on because of how medicated I was. I wasn't in a trance; I was just deluded with faint memories and brief hallucinations. I was either on the most potent cocktail of pain meds which diluted my memory, or physical trauma from the operation, or both. I have no memory of some of the dumb things I did post operatively. I only know what my mother has told me. An example of one of my hallucinations was that I would answer my phone periodically as if someone were calling me. Not only would I answer, but I'd also have a full-blown conversation and then put my phone back down, and I would fade back away into my deep drug-induced slumber.

The medication was a double-edged sword in a myriad of ways. It helped me tremendously in the beginning, with keeping the pain in check. It was so strong that I was sleeping the majority of the time, something that would have been impossible if it wasn't for that pump. When I got slowly got weaned off of the pain killers, time dragged, the pain was more vivid, and the memories weren't getting dulled. Sleep also became impossible unless I administered a couple of doses into my IV.

Some traumatic situations I was presented with in the hospital could not be forgotten. Certain painful memories and soul crushing realizations don't fade away, sadly. They become embedded in your DNA, and it becomes a part of you. Those details are singed into your brain forever. They are placed deep within your cerebral cortex in a place where nothing can be erased. They stick around, replaying over and over again, analyzing every aspect of the trauma. Trying to figure out why it happened and to make sure it will never happen again. From a primal perspective it seems like an ingenious way to evolve—to not be able to forget devastating traumas, to avoid them in the future, keeping that pain real and present in your mind so you are always reminded to be on your toes. Except in this regard, it didn't help that much. Instead, all that was being analyzed was something I couldn't control that I wish I could forget, on a loop over and over again.

## BIG FOOT IN THE PEDIATRIC UNIT

One of the memories that will stick with me forever was how I was treated as a rare specimen of some sorts. I was in the pediatric center of the hospital. This center of the hospital was not accustomed to patients like me. What my parents didn't realize prior to the surgery when they were telling the doctors to put me in pediatrics is that it probably wasn't the smartest choice.

My parents' reasoning made sense beforehand; my mom was put in the gastro unit when she was going through her surgery. She was put next to old dying people, and that experience traumatized her as a young girl. So, my mom figured she would try to prevent me from going through that, but it turns out pediatrics wasn't sunshine and rainbows.

I was a rare sight on the wing of the hospital dedicated to children, the needle in the haystack of the medical world. Like a mythological creature or an urban legend of sorts. I was the Big Foot of the pediatrics unit, and all the doctors and nurses were itching to get a peek at me. Doctors who weren't part of Dr. Gorfine's surgical team would come into the room and prod me. They would come in while I was in my semi-lucid dreamlike state. Floating along, coasting by, I would be not fully comprehending what was going on around me. All of a sudden, the focus lens in my brain snapped into place, and I was fully lucid of what was going on.

They would poke at my bandages and wounds to see it for themselves. I hadn't looked at my wounds at this point. My state of mind wasn't on that level to handle looking at such a horrific site. They would come in and take a look at my abdomen which was covered in blood-soaked gauze from just below my pectorals down to my groin. They would press the gauze with their hands, and some would ask if they could see the main incision site which would require removing my gauze. Some would take it upon themselves to dig around and look for whatever it was they were looking for.

I understand from a medical perspective this is their passion, their absolute burning desire in the world. This is what they get great joy out of doing, this is what fulfills their lives with purpose. I can imagine the jolt that sparked in their brains when they heard there is a patient in their section of the hospital that is fighting a rare genetic condition not many people know about. They wanted to use me to gain insight and knowledge. Coming up to me like an open textbook, waiting to be soaked up by their eager minds that are hungry for another dose of knowledge.

But this isn't a textbook they are approaching; this is another human being. When they poked me, I felt that pain, and I didn't feel just the pain—I felt violated. This was my life they were examining—my suffering, my agony being observed as if it is entertaining, like there is any sort of joy to be had here at this moment. For them, there was a lot to be excited about. For me, there was a lot to feel absolutely petrified about. *Am I a freak? What is so fascinating about me? These people are looking at me as if I have three heads. Am I really that different?*

Isolation is a common thing to feel when you are going through trauma of any sort. If it is a rare shock that not many people can relate to, then it is a whole different beast. The island that you feel stranded on suddenly feels as if you've been launched into space. Lost and floating around an endless vacuum of pain and isolation. The isolation I was feeling deep within my soul was amplified by incidents like this. I couldn't wrap my mind around what was so interesting about me that people were looking at me like I was Big Foot. I had already struggled with the reality of being a patient, and now I had to adjust to being a specimen?

Regardless if it was unintentional, it doesn't excuse this behavior at all. This isn't a smear on doctors or nurses because I know damn well the good they do for people in need. This is more of a call to attention for people in the medical world, that most patients are scared and insecure. *They don't need to be treated as if they are a rarity, even if they are.*

The most upsetting part is that I wasn't in a position to defend myself from the discomfort being inflicted my way. My mom eventually caught a whiff of my displeasure and acted on it immediately. The mama bear protecting her cub instinct had begun to kick in. She was now taking names at the door, and if they weren't part of Dr. Gorfine's team, they were dealt with swiftly and efficiently by my mother. Research time was over, and if you didn't get your chance to see me, the door was forever shut on that situation.

Having my mom in these moments made me reflect on how my hospital trip would have gone if she wasn't there for the overnights. If it was just me, alone in the hospital at night during those eleven days, I can safely say the experience would have been worse and more traumatic if she wasn't there with me. In the beginning days I would not have been able to defend myself or stick up for myself had she not been there. She had to be my voice in certain moments, and I'm very thankful she was there for me—even though I'm sure the hospital staff may have felt differently.

## CHAPTER 6

# THE GOOD...

———

During the beginning of my hospital stay, this one doctor from the surgical team would come in and poke around at my wounds. He had a thick Russian accent, bald head, some scruff for facial hair, but nothing much. Black glasses clung to his face. He was the one who replaced or fixed my bandages.

This is when I started to become hyperaware of my wounds. The first time he came in was still during the period when I was severely drugged up. I was floating in and out of sleep, my dad was at my bedside so it couldn't have been late at night. The room was dark and quiet, until a couple of loud knocks echoed from the door to my bedside.

*Oh no*, I thought to myself. What is about to happen? The door opened; light completely engulfed the dark room that was only illuminated by the TV in the background. He was alone and walked over to my bedside. I started running potential scenarios in my head.

"Alright how are we feeling today, lots of pain? Or only a little bit?" he asked briefly.

"Lots of pain," I whispered out in a hush tone.

"Alright, it's time to change the gauze padding on your stomach. This might hurt, but it needs to be done. I'll try to be quick."

He pulled down the covers of my bed and lifted up my gown. I saw my stomach for the first time. It looked like a war was taking place on my abdomen. There was a large piece of blood-soaked gauze and a green bile colored liquid that started underneath my chest and went all the way down to my groin. To the right of the gauze was my ostomy, which was more gross and shocking to me than anything else going on. It was a clear bag that clung slightly above my hip. It was attached to an opening in the side of my abdomen that had parts of my intestine sticking out. I could see the red nose button that was my small intestine sticking out of my body as the light reflected off its slimy exterior. The contents of what was running through my intestines entered the bag with each pulse.

It pulsated a lot, and with each pulsation I could feel the skin that was pried open for it to stick out, being stretched and ripped apart ever so slightly. The bag was filled with the green, bile colored liquid. Below my bag on each side of my hip were the Jackson-Pratt tubes, or my grenades as I called them.

The Jackson-Pratt tubes were filled roughly to the top with blood and serious fluid. They continued to drain as I stared blankly into the pinkish tinted tube, slowly watching the droplets inch down the tube and drop down creating a ripple in the fluid.

Whenever my grenades filled to the top with my bodily fluids, a nurse would come in and empty them so I could watch the pinkish liquid continue to seep in through the thin tube and into the drain. They hung from my hip and had more or less the same effect as my ostomy. They were pulling on the skin it was connected to.

I wasn't able to see my scar because of all the bandaging, but that would all change when this man changed them. He never had a gentle touch; he would rip off the gauze quickly and when he touched my stomach, he didn't do it with the caution I hoped for. His cold, callus hands would press against my body with force, not giving me anytime to process what was going on. His hands sent a shiver-like reaction from head to toe, which in turn made my abdomen twitch. Whenever my abdomen would twitch, I would enter a world of hurt, and it never took much to make it twitch.

When he ripped the gauze off, I felt the damaged skin and scar tissues on my abdomen pulse with pain. I closed my eyes and bit my tongue. I began to see stars, and after I opened my eyes, I was finally able to get a good look at what was going on below the surface of all those bandages.

Starting a smidge below my belly button was a bloody thick line and if you looked close enough you could see the inside of me. Where my scar was were staples—roughly thirteen of them if I remember correctly. It looked like if the staples weren't there, my stomach would start stretching apart until my insides were on full display. The sight scared me as I saw what the reality of my life was. *Is my stomach going to look like that forever? Am I ever going to be able to take my shirt off confidently again?* The insecurity began to flood my head at an overwhelming rate. I was begging for the numbing effect of my medication to kick back in. Like I said before, some things can't be erased from your memory.

After I got a good look, he was quick to put fresh bandages back on. He finished taping on the new gauze, firmly attaching it to my abdomen.

"Changing the gauze will be standard the first couple days, it won't look like that forever," he said in an attempt to ease the worried look on my face. His effort at consoling felt a bit cold, although it was an attempt, so I guess there's points for trying.

It didn't matter how quick he was; what I saw was etched into my mind, burned into my retinas. After he left that day, I pressed my pain pump begging for the effects of the medicine to kick in as soon as possible so this twisted reality I was living in could be silenced for the moment. This was the start of a routine that would happen about one to two times per day for the first couple days. Once in the beginning and end of the day, he would come in to do the same routine. The first time was definitely the most difficult, to see it on full graphic display—to take it in and look at it. After that, it was still repulsive to look at and it still hurt like hell, but part of me accepted it wasn't going to change. I became numb and callused to it after a while. In the moment I thought this reality would never get any better, so mentally I was defeated.

My nurses were wonderful people and my experience with them was pleasant. I had a handful of nurses and doctors who regularly checked on me but only a few went above the call of duty. My first nurse was a Jamaican woman by the name of Precious. She was a vibrant, loud, and upbeat person, with a smile that could light up Alaska in the polar night. It was hard to not feel comfortable or happy around her. Her caretaking skills were first class, and I felt at ease when she came in.

The nurses had to do a grocery list of rather embarrassing things about me, which made me feel vulnerable. For example, I didn't know how to use my bag or empty it properly. Besides that, I was in no condition to do so. I couldn't sit up in my own bed, so anywhere from two to six times a day the nurses had to empty my colostomy bag for me.

This was probably the most embarrassing thing; there was a bunch but this one really bothered me. Having the bag was a total nightmare. It was a brand-new concept life was throwing at me, a concept I didn't know existed before. I was positive I would hide from everyone until it was off me. I had no idea if I was going to tell my friends, not because I didn't trust them or anything. I couldn't admit it to other people. How can you explain to someone that you go to the bathroom…in a bag attached to your hip where your intestines are sticking out?

Having your independence stripped from your life alters everything about who you are right to the core. Great shame engulfs you when you have to let another person take care of you. It doesn't matter if it is for the better because in the moment, you aren't thinking that way. Accepting I needed others to care for me was especially difficult since I'm a person who prides himself on his independence and values his "me" time. When you have nurses adjusting your catheter, changing your gauze, and emptying your bag, you are doomed to feel insufficient. I couldn't help but feel I needed to apologize to my nurses, which is something I did multiple times.

Something that stuck with me was the response I got from my nighttime nurse Sarah. Sarah was a hard-nosed New Yorker. She had the grit that is associated with natives in the city. She would walk to work at 7 p.m. every night, in time for her to spend the night with me. Sarah was not a quitter, and that oozed out of her personality. She had to take care of relatives with health issues as well. She had a son with an ostomy and did a remarkable job at making me feel like a human being and not a freak. I hope her son realizes how lucky he is to have such a caring mother. As the nurse in the family, she was not only taking care of patients like myself on her night duties, but she was also the caretaker in her apartment. She wasn't new to helping someone take care of their ostomy.

"I'm sorry you have to do this, Sarah," I whispered out to her in a sad tone as she began to change my bag for the first time in the night shift.

"What are you apologizing for?" She cocked her head, looking at me in a confused manner. "This is my job, hon. I'm here to take care of people. You didn't ask for this, but you're still gonna fight through it," she said to me in pep-talk mode. "Besides, this is going to help you in the long run, remember that. It is going to get better, kiddo." She shot a smile at me as she finished clipping the new ostomy on. Then it was off to attend to her other patients. Anyone who had Sarah as their nighttime nurse was a lucky patient.

At that moment, I remember thinking to myself, *She's lying to me.* She was looking at me as if I was strong or brave. I was confused at that notion because I didn't believe I was either of the two. My self-esteem was nonexistent at this point.

For people like me who are incapacitated to the point they can't bathe themselves, some nurses take it upon themselves to give sponge baths to the patient. Precious was one of two nurses who did this, and at first, I didn't want to do it. I didn't want to be that much of a burden to another person that they felt obligated to bathe me. To me it was degrading and a low point in my hospital trip, but she insisted.

That's how she was. She didn't mind doing these things because she cared. I mean some things you can't fake, and genuine kindness is one of them. When you are offering to give patients, who are unable to shower, a sponge bathe, that's an example of genuine kindness. That's something that took a long time for me to fully understand, and it gave me a newfound appreciation for nurses and healthcare workers. I couldn't fathom how much of a burden I thought I was. I pictured myself as this hopeless kid who was so sick he couldn't take care of himself.

She didn't look at me like I was a freak or a misfit. She didn't view me as some burden who was a pain in the butt to deal with. I didn't understand at the time that someone could be so compassionate. I had never experienced compassion like that from a complete stranger before. That was the type of love I was shown from family.

The great people I did encounter at the hospital showed me the better side of the human condition. It is easy to get caught up with the atrocities humans commit on a regular basis. It is easy to forget that with every horrible story we hear about human behavior, there are three more about human compassion. I have seen both sides of the spectrum through-out my battle with FAP.

## CHAPTER 7

# THE BAD AND THE UGLY

———

After a couple of days my nurses and doctors started to push me to move around. I'd been using my pain pump often, and I noticed the nurses giving me attitude about this, as if I was abusing it. I remember after they told me my cheeks began to get flushed with anger. *Who were these people to be giving me attitude when I'm the one in pain? I'm sitting in this bed with tubes coming out of every opening in my body, staples and gauze holding my bloody, swollen stomach together, and they were upset with me for using pain medicine?*

The one doctor with the Russian accent paid me a visit during one of these days when I was being pushed around. When he came in, I could already tell he wasn't pleased. As he was roughly patching up my gauze without being tender to my needs, he managed to make the unpleasant engagement more volatile. After he prodded me and inflicted pain during the changing of my gauze, he asked, "How do you plan on getting out of here if you are not walking around?"

I was stunned and confused. I didn't know how to respond to this man. *Did he actually have the nerve to say that to me?*

"I'm in too much pain to walk around. I can't do it," I responded in a hush tone since speaking still hurt.

"Of course it's going to hurt, but you're never going to get out of here if you don't walk around. You'll never get better either, so unless you enjoy laying in this bed, I suggest you get out of it." Unflinching and without an emotional quiver in his voice, he delivered that line to me cold and uncompassionately.

For the sake of not writing out a bunch of expletives, you can get an idea of how mad I was in this moment.

I was boiling up inside with a white-hot rage that required me to bite my tongue in place, so it didn't start subconsciously hurling four letter obscenities at him. My anger had consumed me to the point where it felt like my face was turning crimson red. I was going to make it my mission to do a hundred laps up and down those hospital halls so he can treat me with a little respect next time we encountered each other.

At that moment in time, I didn't realize this was the nurses and doctor's plan. They were playing poker with me, and in that moment, they trapped me, like Teddy KGB. How do you snap a depressed patient out of a drug-induced haze? You piss them off. Depression makes you submissive. It makes you not care about anything. The only way they could get me to start caring about myself again was to light a fire under me.

*Message received.*

They set gasoline to a massive bonfire which shot right underneath me. The fire was lit, and I was consumed by my anger. I began to channel the anger within to conduct the energy necessary to walk despite the excruciating pain I was in. I suddenly didn't give a second thought about the embarrassing tube hanging out of my butt, I didn't care about the five other tubes that were hanging from other areas of my body. All I could focus on was proving that pompous doctor wrong.

First, I had to maneuver myself up slowly and prepare. Propping myself up into a ninety-degree angle was inflicting serious burning pain up and down my abdomen. I winced for a second and then my dad got ready to help me out.

"Take it slow, son. There's no rush to any of this."

I nodded because the pain was too overwhelming to speak.

I moved my legs slowly toward the edge of the bed as typically this was the hardest part. Swinging them over the edge and getting onto my own two feet was extremely difficult. I had a catheter running down my leg that wasn't in properly, so slight movements created a brutal sensation in the one spot no man wants to get hit. If you don't know what a catheter is, Google it and you'll see what I'm talking about.

I had a tube draining blood from the surgery site coming out of my butt. I looked as if I had a tail underneath my hospital gown. It's bad enough in the hospital they can't give you a decent gown to cover a patient's rear end, with me not only were the goods showing, but I had a present stuck in between my cheeks that by-passers in the hospital got a free show too. Then to add to the circus on my body were the Jackson-Pratt tubes, hanging off each side of my body comparable to a pair of yo-yos.

I was rail thin, incredibly weak, and it looked like the life had been sucked out of me. My face was pasty white, and you could fit a petite women's bracelet around my bicep as if it were a wrist. My cheek bones protruded out of my face as there was no skin or fat to conceal them. My dad helped assist me, and it took about five minutes for me to get out of the bed onto my own two feet. As I stood up on my own, I clutched onto my IV pole and held onto it for dear life. It was my unofficial crutch. If I let go of the pole and tried to walk on my own, I would've fallen to the ground. I was *that* weak.

"Don't be afraid to ask for help. I'll help you walk if you need it," my dad said, concerned.

"It's fine, I want to do this on my own. I want to shut that doctor up," I hissed.

I walked slowly and gingerly out of the room. Walking was more painful than I ever imagined it could be. It was like trying to run a marathon after getting shanked in the stomach. Although I had only walked a maximum of a couple hundred feet, it felt like I had walked about five miles from the aching and throbbing pain pulsing through my body.

Standing up and walking, all these tubes and drains were now being pulled down by gravity. The Jackson-Pratts that hung from my hip were ripping the skin it was connected to. The drain in my butt was doing more or less the same. The catheter was irritating the place where absolutely no man wants to be irritated. My staples and wounds were being dragged down deeper into my skin by gravity. It was awful, but I made it my mission to walk up and down that hall until I passed out.

My life for the next half hour turned into a 1980s training montage, like when Rocky was training in the wood cabin in Rocky IV before he got ready to fight Ivan Drago (if that montage doesn't get you amped up, then nothing will motivate you). I could hear "Hearts on Fire" playing in my head. I channeled my inner Sylvester Stallone as I pushed up and down the hallways.

"That doctor really pissed you off, huh?" my dad said half-jokingly during my walking tirade.

I nodded at him as all my energy was being focused on walking and ignoring the excruciating pain.

"I know you don't believe anything is going to be okay at the moment, but have faith in the process. I trust Dr. Gorfine, and I know you do as well. I remember when your Aunt Maria was going through this," my dad said trying to encourage me.

"I trust him," I said under my breath as I continued to grip my IV pole propelling myself forward. "It doesn't take away the pain or how shitty this is right now."

"I know, it will get better though. Look at everyone in the family now, they all made it out. So, will you."

My dad kept saying we could stop whenever I liked. I didn't want to stop though, not until I didn't have it in me anymore to do it. We weren't stopping until the gas tank was on E, and I was still feeling about half full. After all, would Rocky stop unless he had given it his all? Besides, it would be a pretty rubbish training montage reference if I only walked around for ten minutes then called it a day. That analogy doesn't get busted out for just any instance. The nurses in the hallway saw me going up and down the halls, walking way more than they anticipated me to walk.

As we would pass the nurses, they would give me a look of approval with a slight smirk. Some were a bit more open about the progress I was showing saying the occasional "Good job!" or "Wow you're really getting your steps in today," which were always met with a return smirk from me, then back to the mission at hand. When I finally returned to my room, I think that I had walked for close to an hour. Then I began the effort of getting myself comfortably into bed, which was always a process. Once we got settled into bed,

I pushed my pain pump two times to administer a hard-earned dose of medicine. Next thing I knew, I was out like a light.

The following morning the front doors of my room opened up and in he came, this time with a smile on his face. I could tell my hard work was acknowledged from the previous day. He came over to my bedside to begin the usual routine of changing my gauze.

"If you keep up the hard work like yesterday you'll be out of here in no time. Make sure to keep at it," he said, cracking a smile as he attended to my bandages.

I smiled back at him; in this moment it dawned on me what he was doing. Maybe he wasn't such a miserable doctor, like I had perceived at first. As a matter of fact, it could be looked at courageously what he did. He took on the role of being the catalyst to enrage me for my own benefit, knowing full well I was going to trash him behind his back, as well as curse him out in my head. Even with the change in attitude, his touch was still rough, but I was able to overlook that detail this time around. At least he had a heart underneath his scrubs. Sometimes tough love is needed to get you back on your feet, and I learned to appreciate it. This wouldn't be the last instance of tough love in my life either.

After I started to walk, I was allowed a somewhat regular food diet. For the first couple days all my nutrition was through the IV, but now I could try things like cranberry juice, water, ice cubes, and Jell-O. In the hospital, this was known as the water diet, and I started on it too see how my body would react. After I was introduced to the water diet, I was also informed that I was to limit my pain pump as much as humanly possible and to only use it when I was in dire need of it.

At this point, I was always in pain in the hospital. There was no such thing as not being in pain; it was a matter of how bad it was. The lowest I ever was on a scale of one to ten without medicine was a seven. If I ever got above a seven and I started inching toward extreme, deathly levels of pain, then I was allowed to use the pump. Until I reached that point, I was basically told to suck it up.

Slowly being weaned off the painkillers made things get increasingly bad again. During my first couple days, I didn't have much recollection or memory of what was going on thanks to the medication. I would wake up to get cleaned off, or to get a bandage changed, sometimes I would have a visitor, but I was never coherent. There were times where I would wake up and think to myself, *This isn't bad.* I can press this pump a couple times, take myself to another world and pass out. When I would wake up either half the day was gone, or a new day had started. I assumed I could borderline overdose on pain medicine until I was magically healed.

But, while weaning off, the days dragged by, hours felt like days and days felt like years. I thought I was never going to leave the hospital. The not so bad hospital trip with no memories started to become a nightmare filled with extremely vivid and detailed flashbacks. The traumas I experienced during the coming days I wish I could erase from my brain.

## THE UGLY...

As things got worse for me in the hospital it reached a head within the next day. I was doing well with handling the diet, so they moved me onto bland food. I forget what they were, but they weren't meals. They were barely snacks; they were the next minor step up from the liquids.

Because I was in the pediatric unit and not the gastro unit, they figured since I was digesting the little things okay, maybe I could be treated. So, my dad got Dunkin' Donuts for him and my brother, and they brought me back a little something since it was approved by the nurses and doctors.

My mom was skeptical about this from the start, but she figured maybe things have changed since her surgery and I would be able to process foods quicker. My dad came back with an iced coffee and some munchkins—nothing crazy, stuff I would eat and most people eat pretty routinely. I took a couple sips slowly. After a few more sips I had a munchkin or two and waited to see how it went. That's all I had. It wasn't as if we were being super reckless eating Taco Bell fresh after getting my intestines removed. Or eating Taco Bell in general. At first, I thought I was in the clear and felt fine.

After ten minutes I knew something was about to go terribly wrong and this wasn't a smart decision. I felt nauseous, but this isn't your regular nausea you feel when you're sick. This consumed my body; I got lightheaded and woozy. My stomach was rumbling so loud that my family was able to hear it. Next, I started to have burning pain in my abdomen and I was squirming in agony I felt it coming up my throat and I shot up in my bed.

"Someone get me a bucket or something," I said quickly, sitting upright on the verge of vomiting.

They brought me a big pink bucket, and I leaned over into it. I was dry heaving, but nothing was coming up. The pain going on in my stomach was so intense all I wanted to do was throw up to get it over with. *Boy was I wrong.* What I didn't realize is that when you throw up, you are contracting everything that makes up your core. This might sound like common sense, but I was not anticipating the pain I was about to feel.

The nociceptors in my abdomen were working overtime, firing waves of pain up my spinal cord and to my brain. My sensing pathway was overwhelmed as it dumped the pain on my neurons. My brain was short circuiting with the overload of information being dumped on it. When I finally began throwing up, the pain going on in my abdomen was beyond words.

I was seeing stars as I was throwing up and I thought the staples holding my stomach together were going to pop out one by one. It felt like they were going to rupture, and I thought I was never going to stop puking. I was throwing up this dark green liquid by the gallons.

In the middle of my puking fit Dr. Gorfine walked in on me, and he looked concerned but most of all, displeased. He didn't say anything or yell at anyone, but he wasn't his normal self that day. No dry humor to lighten the mood was coming from him. He didn't stick around to ask me questions, probably because he witnessed me have an extreme vomiting fit which caused me severe pain, so he was able to read the room. This change in his attitude indicated this could have been handled better.

I suspect he caught wind of the nurses and doctors approving of food that wasn't cleared by him yet and wasn't exactly happy with them. Perhaps he was a bit disappointed in me for eating those foods. This is where the pediatric unit was the wrong decision. It wasn't their fault necessarily, they didn't know any better, this wasn't their area of expertise. Not only that but this wasn't Dr. Gorfine's domain, so to speak. He was a little out of his element in this setting and you could tell that was frustrating him a bit. After my puking fit,

I felt I earned the pain pump and a day off from walking, so I pressed the button and knocked out. That concluded my worst day in the hospital.

I always looked forward to the morning visits I would have from Dr. Gorfine. Some days, he was accompanied by his surgical team who were all as helpful and friendly as he was. Other days he came in by himself to talk to me, either way it didn't usually make a difference. If he was with his surgical team, it usually meant they were taking a tube out of me or something of that nature. The reason I enjoyed Dr. Gorfine's visits was his comforting nature.

Everything he said was how it was, no exaggeration for the good or for the worse. He didn't sugar coat things, if it was going to be tough or painful, he told me. If I had overcome the hard part, he would let me know and above all he always added some humor to lighten the mood and make me feel better. The one joke he said after debriefing me on whatever it was we were discussing that day was, "Remember they don't know me around these parts, so it's all about making me look good."

I would chuckle and after I laughed, he would say, "So what's the most important thing?"

"Making you look good," I would say with a smile.

After I said that, he would always laugh and shake it off with, "You know I'm joking."

I always knew he was, and he never had to say it. I'm sure he has an ego and does want me to get better to make him look good. I mean, isn't that what we all want in life? To be respected and admired in our field of choice. Medicine can be a competitive field, especially as a surgeon. It's not a knock on any surgeon if they have a desire to succeed and be the best. After all, patients recovering from *their* work reflects *their* reputations. Not to mention the enormous amounts of stress that come with the profession.

When things got turbulent, however, he never got frustrated with me because his surgery wasn't working so to speak. Some surgeons have the tendency to get frustrated when a patient is lagging in recovery because it will reflect poorly on his work. Dr. Gorfine, while he was always proud of his work (as he should be), never let it get in the way of how he treated his patients. *That's an underrated quality.*

My mom would always hug him and call him our angel on earth for saving our lives and you can tell whenever my mom did this, he was slightly uncomfortable. He didn't view himself that way. I think part of him was a little modest about the role of being some larger-than-life figure in the eyes of my family, or anyone. I respected that aspect of Dr. Gorfine, and I always will. The following morning, he knew I had a tough night and when he came in, he was his prototypical reassuring self.

"Looks like we're doing better today," he said as he walked in.

"Yesterday was a tough one but we're hanging in there today," said my mom.

"I know, I appeared to have come at a bad time yesterday. To ease your mind, everything that happened yesterday was normal and expected. Maybe eating the food wasn't a great idea, but it was going to happen eventually. The stuff you were throwing up was bile; it needed to come up. That's why you felt sick, and I would imagine you feel considerably better today," he explained to me thoughtfully.

"Yes, today is much better than yesterday. I'm scared to eat because of that though. The pain from throwing up was too much on my abdomen. I can't do it again," I said, concerned.

"There shouldn't be more throwing up; I suspect that it all came out yesterday. It should be smooth sailing moving forward."

"Well that's a relief."

He looked at me and my mom with a thoughtful expression, smiled, and began to tell a story: "I want you to know that what you're going through is something I'd never be able to handle. I'm the worst patient, and the only major operation of any sort I ever had was my wisdom teeth!"

"Sounds like you're quite fortunate if that's all you've had done," I replied.

"Extremely, which is the point I'm making. That's all I ever had done to me, and I was a total baby. I sit here and see what you've been through, and you're not making a fuss about it. Meanwhile, I was making a fuss out of my wisdom teeth."

I smiled, I appreciated why he was telling me this. Although I don't think he realized that the only reason I wasn't making a fuss is because I was so weak. *I couldn't make a fuss even if I wanted to and believe me I did.*

"I guess that makes me stronger than you," I decided to joke back with him.

He smiled as he grabbed his clipboard before he left to make his other rounds. "It appears that way, doesn't it?" He then exited the room to spread his charm to the rest of his patients.

That story would always make me chuckle and put a smile on my face. It made me feel like I wasn't a total wimp. It made me feel like maybe I was strong.

# CHAPTER 8

# TRAUMA

———

Time was dragging as I was trapped in bed suffering in my own misery. The reality of my life was beginning to dawn on me, and the pain was hitting extra hard. On social media, I saw all of my friends and classmates having the time of their lives prior to them departing for what was next for them. And where was I?

I was in a hospital bed in New York City, suffering—suffering unspeakable things none of those people will ever experience. Then began the grieving for me. I began to blame the world for everything that was happening.

*If there's a God, why is he doing this to me? What did I do to deserve this? Why was I being punished?*

I was angry at the world and I couldn't make sense of it. Everything had come crashing down on me. Every raw emotion you experience after having your life changed by a major altering event smacked me in the face and knocked me down. I was feeling left out watching everyone continue onto their next chapter, while I was stuck.

As I sat in a hospital bed in agonizing pain, intentionally weaning myself off the only thing that was bringing me peace, my mind started to deteriorate. This is when my real challenge began. Physical pain sucks, and there is no doubt about that. Mental pain is in a league of its own. Combine the two together at the same time, and you've got what truly feels like an impossible mountain to climb.

## THE MENTAL HEALTH STRUGGLE

When you suffer emotional trauma there is no yearly checkup to get yourself fixed, but we have a yearly physical for our bodies. The damage done to your psyche if you suffer emotional trauma never goes away over time if left unchecked and can cause a myriad of issues down the road, such as involuntary outbursts of shame, guilt, and anger.[11] When you experience trauma, the simple memory of that event can mess with your psychological well-being. Memories of physical pain don't bring that same level of physical discomfort back to you like emotional pain can (and let's be thankful for that, or else I would never be without pain).

This is why PTSD is a major problem for anyone who has experienced something traumatic. For veterans returning from battle, it's hard to adjust to normal civilian life after facing life or death scenarios on a daily basis. Just like it's hard for someone who's been abused emotionally or sexually to let their guard down to another person.

These issues don't only affect the individual; they can also affect the people around them. It is important for society to understand that sometimes people's actions toward you aren't the entire picture, and we should refrain from spreading rumors, judging, or further adding to whatever stress they might be dealing with. Trauma is subjective, however,

---

11    Lawrence Robinson, "Emotional and Psychological Trauma," HelpGuide. org, Accessed January 19, 2021.

as others can experience certain stressful situations that don't trigger PTSD or stress disorders in general. Trauma has different definitions for everyone, and because something might not traumatize you per se, it could be wreaking havoc on someone else. Maybe they are having trouble dealing with it and you see it being expressed outwardly, challenge yourself to dig a little deeper and not judge at face value.

We live in the modern world, so mental health has to be improving compared to generations past, right? Unfortunately, this is not the case, with suicide being the tenth overall cause of death in the United States claiming over 48,000 lives according to the Centers for Disease Control and Prevention leading causes of death report.[12] To give this number some perspective, that is more than twice the amount of homicide victims (18,830) in the same time period.[13] For people in my age bracket, ten to thirty-four years of age, suicide is the second leading cause of death with only unintentional injuries above it.[14] Unintentional injuries include drowning, motor vehicle accidents, firearms, and burn victims.

As citizens of the United States, we constantly hear about the problem of gun violence because of the number of lives it claims every year. We are even more horrified when a mass shooting happens, and rightfully so. It doesn't appear we show the same signs of urgency for our dramatically increasing suicide rates, which now dominate the homicide numbers. If homicides are considered a major problem in our

---

12  "Suicide Statistics," National Institute of Mental Health, US Department of Health and Human Services, January 2021.

13  Ibid.

14  Ibid.

country—and it is—I wonder when mental health might get the same treatment.

With all these different outlets of information at our disposal every day, what could possibly explain this epidemic we are seeing? According to preliminary results from an ongoing study funded by the National Institutes of Health, brain scans of adolescents who are heavy screen users (smart phone, video games, tablets) look different than those adolescents who used less screen times.[15] In the first round of testing scans of children that reported daily screen usage of seven hours showed premature thinning of the brain cortex, the outermost layer that processes information from the physical world.[16] If you think seven hours of daily screen time is something you can't achieve because it seems a bit ridiculous, I advise you to check your screen time usage in your iPhones. The answer might shock you. Especially as we live in a world dependent on our black mirrors because of the coronavirus pandemic.

These studies are ongoing and are subject to change. The results of this information aren't conclusive yet. We have only been living with social media for a decade, and in a lot of ways we are acting as real time tech guinea pigs. There is a lot of good to be had from social media, especially in the year 2020 as we have been reliant upon our technology to be in contact with our friends and loved ones. Social media should be making us feel more connected, right? According to one experiment, people who were randomly assigned to give up Facebook for a week ended that time period happier, less

15    Lisa Lee, "NIH Study Probes Impact of Heavy Screen Time on Young Brains," BloombergQuint, December 11, 2018.

16    Ibid.

lonely, and less depressed than those who kept their Facebook accounts.[17] In addition to this information, several longitudinal studies indicated that screen time leads to unhappiness, but unhappiness doesn't lead to more screen time.[18]

This isn't to say that social media and technology are the sole reasons we ended up in this predicament, but it would be foolish to not realize it is playing a role. Other factors could be because of the fast-paced world we live in. Perhaps it's a culmination of issues that have been piling on top of each other to lead to this boiling point. Whatever we decide to point the finger at and blame, the bottom line is three in five Americans consider themselves lonely, a seven-point increase from 2018.[19] Seventy-nine percent of Gen Zers surveyed reported feeling lonely, along with 71 percent of millennials and 50 percent of baby boomers.[20] Some people reading this book might be thinking to themselves, *Pfft, who cares? Everyone gets lonely, right?* Perhaps this statistic will make you consider the dangers of loneliness. According to published research, being disconnected and lonely poses danger equivalent to smoking fifteen cigarettes a day and was more predictive of early death than the effects of air pollution or

17  Morton Tromholt, "The Facebook Experiment: Quitting Facebook Leads to Higher Levels of Well-Being," Cyberpsychology, behavior and social networking, US National Library of Medicine, November 1, 2016.

18  Jean Twenge, "What Might Explain the Current Unhappiness Epidemic?" Ladders, April 23, 2020.

19  Carrie M Jones, "The Loneliness Epidemic Revisited: A 2020 Update," CMSWire.com, February 19, 2020.

20  Ibid.

physical inactivity.[21] So, unless you're already chain smoking a pack of cigs a day, we should all be aware of this. We are social creatures after all.

The point of me throwing this information at you isn't to put a face to the boogeyman that explains why so many of us are feeling lonely and upset these days. It's to shed some light on the causes that we currently know of, and to correct these behaviors if applicable—behaviors like learning how to use social media and technology properly. We don't take social media etiquette classes in high school (although that should be added to the curriculum if you ask me), and it clearly poses dangers we didn't quite understand when these inventions were first concocted. It's necessary to know that comparing your life on social media to others isn't healthy. I would know; I spent a whole summer in the hospital and on my couch basking in the misery of comparing my sad existence to all these seemingly happy people. I consider myself one of the lucky ones because not everyone makes it out of my circumstances, which is evident with our current suicide numbers. It took me until just recently, and I'm still learning every day that what you see online isn't reality.

Lastly, if there is anything we can learn from the dumpster fire that was the year 2020, it is to be better to one another. It's easy to treat life as a competition, with social media as your platform to boast your accomplishments in the faces of your peers. Perhaps you want to gloat and make others feel stupid for doubting you. The bottom line is, we are all human and we all crave *positive* social relationships.

---

21   Jenny Anderson, "Loneliness Is Bad for Our Health, Now Governments around the World Are Finally Tackling It," Quartz, October 9, 2018.

## MEETING DIMITRI

I didn't have a roommate for my first couple of days in the hospital. I was pretty happy with having my own space so no one else was a witness to what was happening to me besides my family and the staff at the hospital. When I was informed I would be having a roommate, I was upset, and it added to the frustration I was experiencing.

In entered the room a young boy who was being called Dimitri by staff at the hospital; they seemed to be familiar with who he was. He was slightly taller than me, when I wasn't hunched over and could stand up properly. He had a buzz cut similar to mine, and we had the same attire which was Mount Sinai's lovely white hospital gown with the horrible design of leaving the butt totally exposed.

"Hey Dimitri, how are we feeling today?" asked a doctor as he was surrounded by what I presumed was his surgical staff.

Dimitri propped himself up in the bed. "Good, but I don't want to be here. Can't I go home?" He didn't seem to perceive what was happening to him on this day, which I found a little odd because they seemed to know him all too well.

His mother sat in the chair next to his bedside, similar to mine. She looked tired, and a bit nervous. "We have to do this, Dimitri. Mommy is going to be right by your side, you hear me?" she said, rubbing his arm in a consoling manner.

"Yeah Dimitri, the pacemaker is going to make you feel better. It's going to help you," the doctor said, explaining the procedure slowly and in an extremely vanilla manner. I didn't know what a pacemaker was at the time, and his description didn't help much, but I think that was done intentionally.

"I just...want to be normal," he said in a defeated tone, slumping his shoulders down.

The doctors and his mother looked a bit upset at his comments; I know it was tough for my father to hear.

"Dimitri, after we get this done, you will be normal, bud. We promise." The doctor fished for a segue to perk his mood up. "What do you want to do when your finally out of here?" he asked.

Dimitri's frown quickly turned into a slight smirk as he enthusiastically said, "I want to be a construction worker!" He rubbed his chin in thought. "I wouldn't mind working here seeing you guys all the time. Y'all are my friends, right?"

"Of course, Dimitri, did you get the impression we weren't?" the doctor chuckled.

"No, I know, I know. I could be a rapper too, ya know! I could freestyle for you guys or beat box. I can do that too." His mind skipped from one idea to the next, rattling off ideas of his life when he finally breaks free from these hospital walls.

What I didn't realize initially is that Dimitri had a stroke, which left irreversible damage to parts of his brain. Dimitri was actually older than me; I was eighteen at the time and Dimitri was in his twenties, although I'm not sure of his exact age. The damage done to his brain left him with the personality of a child, with emotional outbursts, mood swings, and certain cognitive disabilities. Dimitri was far from being a totally dependent individual though. You would think a person who suffered a stroke and has cognitive damage wouldn't be able to rap and beat box in a creative manner. The energy he exhibited and his enthusiasm to fit in showed me he not only wanted to be independent, but he could be. Perhaps he might need some help, as I don't know the complexity of his situation, but he seemed to have a good quality of life given his circumstances, which made me happy.

He certainly had a vibrant personality, and a mostly positive attitude given his situation. The pacemaker going into Dimitri's heart was to hopefully prevent future cardiovascular issues as he had sickle cell anemia, a fate far worse than mine, which made me reflect internally on what I was dealing with.

When I fell asleep that night, my dad had some one-on-one time with Dimitri, where he started a conversation with my dad.

"Are you Michael's dad?" Dimitri asked as he propped himself up in bed.

"Yes, I am Michael's dad," my dad answered politely.

In a concerned tone, Dimitri asked, "Is he going to be okay? It seems he's in a lot of pain."

The genuine concern of Dimitri pulled on my dad's heartstrings.

"He's been through a lot...but he's going to be okay." He composed himself some more. "He's talkative usually, but he's hurting right now. I know he'll warm up; give him time."

"If you don't mind me asking sir, what's wrong with him?" Dimitri asked looking concerned and eager to find out.

"Well, it's pretty complicated, but to put it simply, he had to get his large intestine removed."

His eyes widened, and his jaw dropped a bit. "Woah... really? The whole thing? There's nothing left?"

"Nope, nothing left. Pretty crazy, huh?"

Dimitri continuing to look shocked. "Wow, that must've hurt. I can see why he doesn't want to talk."

"Let's see how he feels when he wakes up. I think he'll be in a more pleasant mood. Hopefully."

The next morning when I had awoken, it was time to walk around. The curtain that usually divided the room was pulled back, so once I began stirring around, Dimitri saw I was awake. As I slowly gathered myself together, fighting the pain associated with propping myself up, I saw Dimitri's eyes light up with a look asking for permission to speak. I looked back at him in a friendly manner, which was all he needed.

"Hi, Mike! I don't know if you remember me, but I'm Dimitri, your roommate," he said with a smile.

"Hey, Dimitri," I winced in pain as I swung my legs over the side of the bed. "I remember a little bit." I paused to catch my breath for a moment.

"I was talking to your dad! He's a nice guy."

"Runs in the family," I said trying to crack a smile.

"He told me a little bit about what you're going through. You're strong for walking around after all that, y'know? I couldn't do it that's for sure."

"It's not my choice unfortunately. I have to do it to get better." At this point, I had both legs swung over the side of the bed, my trusty IV pole positioned by my side.

"Doing what the doctors tell you is never easy, but it's for the better. I always listen to the doctors here; they are the best. They know me if they didn't already tell you. Plus, I work in the cafeteria when they're not fixing me up."

I smiled and nodded. "That's awesome that you have a job here."

He saw my struggles in that room, and I saw his too. Seeing each other's pain and suffering created mutual respect between the two of us. Later on, when I would go through my second surgery, it became apparent how much he respected me after the days we shared in the hospital.

\*\*\*

My second surgery was roughly three months after my initial takedown surgery, the morning of my next step in the process my parents headed to the cafeteria in the hospital to get breakfast to pass the time as they were anxious for my well-being. They told me they were saying a prayer at the table and moments later, Dimitri, who was working in the cafeteria that day, recognized my parents and came up and talked with them. He was so excited to see them.

Dimitri waved his hands and approached my parents as they waived back. "What brings you guys here again? Michael isn't in here, is he?" His tone switched from excited to concerned.

My dad looked up at Dimitri. "Today is the day of his second operation; it's two parts."

Dimitri put his hands on his hips. "Well, he's going to be fine. I know he is. He made it out the first time, and so did I. If I can do it, so can he."

My mom uncrossed her hands from her praying position. "Thank you, Dimitri. That's sweet of you." My dad nodded, agreeing with my mom.

My mom perked up. "This is our sign, Dimitri!"

He looked confused at my mom. "Sign?"

"We came down here to say a prayer for Michael before his second surgery, Dimitri. We were sitting here praying for a sign things would be okay. Then you approached us. What are the odds after all these months?"

It clicked for Dimitri what my mom was saying, and his face lit up with a smile. "Sounds like a sign to me. I'll keep Mike in my prayers. I hope he does well down the road."

"Thank you, Dimitri, it means a lot to us. When Michael wakes up, we'll tell him we ran into you. I'm sure he'll be happy to hear that."

Oddly enough, we never got into contact with Dimitri after that encounter. We had a lot going on in our lives, as I'm sure he did as well. After all these years a part of me is curious about how he is doing. I hope he is doing well like I am. I hope he is still able to live a full and fun life. There was an article about him on the internet where he met Nick Cannon. I remember him telling us this in the hospital one day, and we looked it up. I have tried finding the article since then but haven't had any luck. It would be nice to see how he's doing. The timing of the whole situation was peculiar, and I found it interesting to this day; it's funny how some things work out.

Having Dimitri as a roommate taught me a great deal of wisdom in my life. He made me realize people out there do have it worse than me and you have to enjoy the life you have no matter how flawed it may be. Who is to say what a normal life is? Even if it is "normal," you have to be thankful for what you got all the time.

No one is free from trauma in life, it happens to all of us eventually. Each trauma is different from the next, and how we react to it is up to the individual. Adversity is the one constant in life we will all face at some point. We will struggle. We will suffer. This is to be expected as no life is free from pain. How we choose to handle this is what ultimately defines our existence.

# PART III

# CROSSROADS

# CHAPTER 9

# DISCHARGED

———

To finish off my stay in the hospital following my first surgery, one of the realities I had to accept was learning how to clean and change the bag on my own. It was a requirement for me to be able to leave, so I absolutely had to do it. The ostomy nurse came into the hospital that day, and I had to participate. The thought of it put me into a mental spin cycle. I was embarrassed, self-conscious, and I didn't want to accept my situation. I thought someone else would do it for me till my recovery was over after three months. That reality was not going to happen.

I had to learn to get my own freedom, but I didn't want to accept it. This wasn't supposed to happen in the breakdown given to me before the surgery. I was told the odds favored this wouldn't happen, and yet here I was. Not only was I not supposed to have it, but three months seemed close to an eternity. I told myself I would sit home and do nothing for three months. I was ashamed of who I was; I didn't want anyone to know or see me in this condition. I was rail thin; you could see my ribs, and I had this horrible bag on me. I especially didn't want to go out in public. The thought of it leaking was a terrifying possibility, a whole disaster in and of its own. *What do I do then?*

These were questions I never imagined myself having to ask. As I lay in the hospital bed, the ostomy nurse came in to pay me a visit and give me a lesson in taking care of my stoma.

"Hello Michael, I'm the ostomy nurse with the hospital." She was upbeat and in her right hand was a stuffed animal, a small otter with a big smile on his face. On the right side of the otter's abdomen was an ostomy bag and a name tag above his chest that read "Ollie."

I nodded. I knew what was about to happen, and I was clearly not thrilled.

"Sorry he's not happy at all about this situation. He doesn't want to clean it or accept he has to." My mom jumped in with concern for the nurse.

"Not to worry, Michael, it's normal. This is something drastically new. I'm here to let you know this isn't as terrible as you believe it is. It's only temporary, and it's helping you heal. This is going to a distant memory before too long."

It was the truth, though I didn't realize it at the moment. Turns out having the bag might have saved my quality of life. When you get a J-pouch, there are two routes typically: the removal of the colon and the construction of the pouch, which I had already gone through. Some practices, after the total removal and construction of the pouch, don't give patients a stoma and let the waste resume course with no time to heal. In my diminished capacity, it is easy to see why this option wouldn't have worked out for me, and why my particular surgeons stopped doing this. The point of the bag, which the nurse pointed out no matter how much I hated it, was to give my intestines time to heal before putting them back to work. It was necessary. The time to heal is probably why I recovered as well as I did.

We have a family friend who got the one-part J-pouch operation under a different surgical staff, and it was an uphill battle for her for more than a year. Not only was it an uphill battle, but she didn't have the gene run in her family. She was one of the unlucky 25 to 30 percent who get the gene spontaneously. Her recovery took about a year longer than mine, and for a little while they were concerned about her health. At the bare minimum, I would've had a much longer recovery. I have a ton to thank my ostomy for now, including the quality of life I have today. If I had the one-part operation, I would've been going to the bathroom twenty plus times a day, while being in an incapacitated state. To this day, my family and I celebrate the blessing in disguise the bag was. I certainly didn't see it that way in the moment. *It's funny how some things play out.*

The ostomy nurse was talking to me, using Ollie to cheer me up, but I wasn't interested in talking back. Ollie the Otter sitting comfortably in the palm of her hand was a gesture to make me smile. Her gesture didn't work, and it wasn't her fault. I wasn't in a good place mentally to appreciate her kindness. Looking back on it, it was a cute gesture, and she was a wonderful woman. My anger and distaste weren't directed at her, she did nothing wrong. It was more so directed at life in general.

My parents expressed their gratitude for what she was doing. I suppose that was enough; maybe one day, she will read this and understand I was grateful for her kind nature.

As my time started to dwindle down in the hospital, it meant getting me in shape to leave, which included removing the Jackson-Pratt tubes. When I first discovered my "grenade tubes" hanging from my waist, I wondered to myself, *How the hell are they going to get these out?* I knew what the answer was, but I wasn't quite ready to accept that reality yet.

The day they were ready to take the first tube out, Dr. Gorfine's surgical team all participated. Three doctors came in while I was in the middle of a visit from my Aunt.

"Hello Michael, hello everybody, how are you all doing today?" exclaimed a young nurse from Gorfine's surgical team.

"We are doing better today; he's got company from some good people to keep his spirits up," my mom said with a smile.

"Yeah, they aren't so bad. They make things a little easier," I said, cracking a smile.

"Well, today we have to remove one of the tubes that are hanging from your waist. You can either get one done for today, or you can get them both taken out; it is up to you."

*Shit.* I was dreading this day, and I didn't want to have it done with company here.

"That's today…" My heart rate increased, and I looked around hoping someone would say it was a mistake. "Can that wait? We have to do it today?" I pleaded to the nurse hoping I would get a break.

"Well unfortunately, no," the nurse said as her expression changed from jovial to somber. "But this means you're closer to getting out of here. That is what you want, right?"

*Easy to say when the tube isn't being yanked from your body.*

I was in full panic mode and looked to my mom and aunt for guidance.

"It's okay, Marlene. I'll talk to him," my aunt whispered to my mom, giving her a break from the constant stress she'd been facing taking care of me on a daily basis.

"Is this going to hurt Aunt Re?" I asked nervously.

"We aren't the type to lie in this family, and I'm not going to lie to you," she said, biting her lip in preparation to break the bad news in a subtle way. "It is going to hurt, but it is going to be quick. I promise you that. You have to count to five, you can hold me and your mom's hand. Take all the pain out on us, it will be over quickly." She slipped me her hand for permission to squeeze away.

"This is going to hurt bad isn't it?" I asked, looking up at the nurse.

She looked back at me, eyes wide, mouth sewn shut. Her facial expression said it all, then she nodded subtly. "I've done this a handful of times. Typically the patients are in pain afterward."

*Here we go*, I thought to myself. There isn't much I could do about it now; I had to bite the bullet.

"Okay, let me get ready."

I closed my eyes and squeezed my mom and my aunt's hands.

"Are you ready, Michael?" asked the nurse, waiting for the final verdict.

"Yes, as ready as I could possibly be."

"Okay…three…two…one…"

And it began. The one male doctor on the surgical team cut the stitches holding the tube in place. He then proceeded to *rip* the tube out of my body. I could feel the tube unwind itself inside of my body as it funneled to the outside world. It was a solid five seconds of the doctor tugging this thing out of me, but it felt like an eternity. I squeezed my mom and aunt's hands with all my might. I began to see stars as I squinted my face waiting for it to be over. I held my breath as I was in utter shock at the pain that was going on in my body. The feeling of the tube unwinding inside of me and making its way out is something I will never forget, and something I can't describe properly to give it the full scale of how painful it was.

"Okay, all done!" exclaimed the male doctor.

I sat there grunting and breathing heavily, trying to get a grip on reality again.

"So," the doctor paused studying my body language, realizing the amount of pain I was in, "I'm assuming you want to wait on getting the other one out?"

*Correct assumption.*

"I can't do that again…not today," I whispered in total agony.

"Okay, that's understandable. We'll be back tomorrow to get the other one out." Then the surgical team went on with their way.

Part of me was relieved the other damn tube wasn't going to be ripped out of me and I'd get a day's reprieve. This feeling of relief was bittersweet, however, as I realized that come tomorrow, I would experience that same dreadful pain.

"It's okay kiddo, it's over with now. You did it," Aunt Re groaned jokingly.

"You almost broke me and your aunt's hand, but it's okay," my mom said.

"I'm sorry. It was so painful."

"It's okay sweetie, I'm only kidding. I know it was. You can press the pump. You've earned it," my mom said reassuringly as she massaged the hand that I had been holding.

On the way in the room was a much-needed and pleasant surprise. My grandma and grandpa arrived for a visit as the surgical team was leaving.

"Hey, buddy!" my grandpa said as he came around the corner with his typical jovial smile.

"He's in a lot of pain right now, Dad. Give him a couple of minutes, and he will be ready for a visit," Aunt Re said to my grandparents.

"No, they can stay." I tried to get control of my breathing. "Give me a minute, and I'll be good."

My mom was a bit shocked at me being so open to visitors after something so painful. "Oh okay, come on in then. Give him a minute so he can talk again."

After I got a minute to compose myself, my grandparents took a seat next to my bed.

"He had one of the grenade tubes pulled out just before you got here," my aunt explained to help get them up to speed.

"Oh, we know those tubes very well, Michael. Everyone in the club had to get those stupid tubes removed," my grandma said, taking hold of my hand.

"You and your mom had those tubes as well?" I was slightly confused because we had different surgeries.

"We may have all had different surgeries from different times, but those tubes have never changed. They hurt for all of us; it wasn't just you. Although from what your Aunt Re has said, you definitely handled it better than her."

"Oh, he definitely handled it better than me. He didn't let out a *fuck* or a *shit* or nothing. No cursing, no crying like I did. He closed his eyes and toughed it out."

"Although I would like to say he almost broke our hands," my mom said with a laugh.

"Oh, shut it, you two will live," my grandma sarcastically snarked at my mom and aunt.

"He knows we're only joking," my aunt said, grinning. "Besides if we can't joke with him then who can?"

*Good point.*

"I guess that makes me feel a little better knowing I handled it the best," I said, feeling proud of myself.

"That's because you're the man of the club—you grit your teeth and ask, 'What's next?'" my grandpa said, adding a chuckle to the conversation.

"I learned my toughness from the toughest guy there is." I pointed at my grandpa in a goofy, stereotypical, macho way.

"You sure did, buddy."

"You want to hear a story about what I had to go through when I was diagnosed?" my grandma asked me.

Surprised, it dawned on me that I hadn't actually heard her full story before.

"Absolutely," I quickly said.

"My sister and I were guinea pigs for our surgery. Aunt Ronnie was number twelve in the world to be operated on for our unique new method, and I was number thirteen, It was back in the '70s when medicine was different from what it is now. I still had the grenade tubes like what you have, and the tube in the butt wasn't fun either. We also had an NG tube, which went in our nose and down to our stomachs."

"Ouch, that sounds…awful."

"Oh, it was. Your mother hated it more than I did when she had her surgery. Anyway, you remember when you threw up that green stuff?"

"How could I forget," I said in a disgusted, sarcastic voice.

My grandma stuck out her tongue in a playful way laughing at my sarcasm. "Well back in the day, the NG tube was used to suck that stuff out of our stomach. We didn't puke it up or let it come up naturally. They had to stick those tubes in our nose and suck that stuff out of us. Me and your Aunt Ronnie were roommates as we went through all of this. Any time they did something to her or vice versa, we would have time to prepare for what was going to happen next. The truth is, it was so unbelievably different than today. They didn't know what to do with us back then, but now they do. It's much better today than it was, and I know you will come out of this a better, stronger person," she finished, looking at me with pride in her eyes.

I was entranced hearing her so calmly explain the horrors she had gone through.

"I never knew any of that, Gram. I never knew anything had happened to you until this past year when I got the news of my test results. Same with Mom and Aunt Re; I never knew."

"Well, because look at us all now. We are all healthy, and life is good. You will be healthy one day too. It will take time. You have us to help you get through the tough times."

Finding out they went through the same experiences as me and some even worse experiences opened a new perspective for me. I never knew any of this about my grandma, and you would never guess it based on how my grandma lived her life. My grandma was always the fun grandma who could keep up with her grandchildren's youthful energy. Never once showing an indication any of these things happened to her. *If she went through all that and was able to live life so fully and gracefully, what's the excuse for me?*

After everything I had just been through, their visit was like having the sun come out and evaporate the clouds. I felt at ease knowing I wasn't alone. My grandparents and my aunt proved to be a genuine comfort to me. The conversation then shifted to a new topic while my dad turned to the Yankee's game on the TV. It was nice for "the club" to be there to support me. Sharing similar experiences we all went through during our different surgeries created a bond with us. We were already bonded as family, but this added a new dimension to our relationship. I always had the utmost respect and love for my grandma, my aunt, and my mom. The club added a new level. The ultimate support group.

Our condition is super rare, on top of being genetic. You don't run into people with this condition, ever. It gave us an outlet to share our experiences with one another. It opened up a new side to my grandma, my aunt, and my mom. I knew we all shared the same condition, but what I had not realized until this day was we all battled things differently. Some worse than others, but we all battled. We all experienced the lows that are associated with having FAP.

My grandma and my mom had it worse than me and my aunt. My grandma spent months in the hospital, while undergoing experimental treatments in the years in-between surgeries. Me and my aunt only spent around eleven days. *Only eleven days.* Both my mom and my grandma got operated on when they were sick and a little older than me and my aunt. My grandma and my mom both learned from the mistakes of the past to operate on us as soon as possible. My aunt and I benefited from Father Time being on our side. The blueprint on how to take care of this illness as best as possible was already laid out, and the trial and error to get the end result were conducted by my mom and my grandma. There were no experimental treatments or blips in the hospital that led to me staying for months—*thank God.* I would learn more about my family's medical history as time progressed.

**HOME BOUND**

The next day, the surgical team visited me again. They took out the other tube, and it was as equally painful as the first time. I also had to get a tube cut and removed from my butt as well. That tube was only embarrassing, not exactly painful physically.

One of my final nights in the hospital, I had a nurse think it was time to take out my catheter, but it turns out I couldn't pee on my own, and I still needed the catheter. I had to pee at an emergency level and when I released nothing was happening. No matter how hard I tried to push, nothing would happen, and the pressure got worse. I had to go—probably the worst I ever had to go in my life. I was pushing the limits of my bladder. It was awful. I could feel my bladder stretching, begging for a release and no sign of relief was in sight. I was genuinely scared my bladder was going to perforate.

My mom rushed to get the nurse in there and she had trouble getting the catheter back in. Poking a catheter in the wrong way down there is a nightmare situation for any guy. I don't need to go into vivid detail as to why; you can let your imagination play with that one.

It was put in wrong about three times and it took about ten minutes for them to get it in the right way. After it finally went in the right way, I was able to relieve myself, but my man area was a little tender from all the poking and prodding. If I thought this situation was embarrassing, boy was I in for a rude awakening come nighttime...

When you get too much fluid with the bag it fills up quickly, but no one told my mom or me this. So, we fell asleep and the next morning no nurses had checked on me, and the bag had burst. It was everywhere and it was an absolute nightmare, as you could probably imagine. After the nurses cleaned it up and after we got myself cleaned up, my mom and I cried. The embarrassment and pain hit a peak with me.

After the cry, we wound up having a little vent session. "Talk to me please, Michael. Let me know what's going on.

You can vent, you can cry, you can tell me anything, I want to know what's going on in your head," she said, as she wiped her eyes.

I was hesitant to answer her honestly. Did she actually want to know what I was thinking? After a brief hesitation, I poured out my emotions.

"Well...I'm not happy." I was reluctant to say the next part. "I wasn't supposed to have this stupid bag and now I'm stuck with it. I don't want to take care of it; I don't want to go out in public. I don't have the willpower to try and move past this. It's too much."

My mom's eyes were red and teary. She held my hand.

"It hasn't been easy for me either. For the last couple months, I haven't had a good night's sleep. The truth is, I can't sleep." Now she looked hesitant to say the next part. "I keep feeling so guilty I gave you this. It's all my fault, I gave you my shitty gene and I try to pretend I've been okay, but I haven't been." Tears now flowing, she wiped her eyes.

My eyes began to get red as well. I didn't enjoy hearing her blame herself.

"It's not your fault, Mom; don't blame yourself. I don't want you to feel guilty. That isn't my goal here. You wanted me to talk, and I'm telling you what's on my mind."

"I know you're not, but hearing you say how upset you are and watching you go through this in the hospital firsthand is too much—especially knowing I could have prevented this; it's my gene. It's not your father's; not anyone to blame but myself."

I cut her off before she could continue. "Don't blame yourself. Please."

There was a brief pause where we were both crying, and then she continued.

"This is why I spend the nights with you in the hospital. It's the absolute least I can do. I gave you this; I can make sure you are not going through it alone. That's what I hated the most when I was going through this, being on my own. When you sleep, I would sneak off into the game room when you had no visitors."

I was a bit confused by her last statement.

"Why would you sneak off there?"

"I would sit in there and cry. I didn't want to cry in front of you to look weak or scare you. I would sit there, cry and blame myself for putting you through this." We both began to cry.

The end of the hospital trip had taken its toll on the both of us, leading us to spill our guts and confess the feelings bottled up inside. I felt awful hearing my mom say how guilty she felt and seeing her so upset wasn't easy. The emotional rollercoaster of the situation had finally reached its peak, and we could no longer hide our emotions.

It definitely helped to have that conversation with my mom. There had been a bit of an elephant in the room leading up until that point. Neither of us had confessed the guilt and stress we had been feeling with each other. It was only a matter of time until it boiled over. It hurt to hear her say how guilty she felt about this whole situation. It was necessary in the long run, however, to know how my mother was feeling in these moments.

After that night, I spiked a fever. The fever made my stay in hospital about a day or two longer and added unnecessary pain. I was already weak and fatigued, and the fever amplified that more. With me not being able to move, I was being prodded with these shots two to three times a day. They were for multiple reasons that I honestly forget now.

At this point, I didn't care much about what was being done to me. I would sit in the bed, and they would come in to do what had to be done. Take a tube out, stick a needle in me, change gauze padding…What else could be done to me that could be worse than what I have already endured? I got around two to three shots per day on each arm and by the end of my stay, once I got home, I looked comparable to a drug addict. With my skinny physique, bruised veins up and down my arms from needle injections, I wasn't looking particularly cute.

My last day in the hospital was a happy event for everyone else but me. The fighting was still far from over for me, and I knew that. Leaving the hospital didn't mean much; it meant my battle was being moved from the hospital to my house. Things didn't get much better for a good little while when I got home, and it was what I expected.

My last day in the hospital I weighed in at about 130 pounds. I was down thirty-five pounds from when I came in and I looked a shell of myself. I had to be assisted to put clothes on, and I needed help with someone to walk around or stand up. I had to be put in a wheelchair and whisked out of the hospital; I couldn't leave on my own will.

When I got wheeled outside for the first time in weeks, the mid-summer sun began to absorb into my pasty, vitamin D-deprived skin. The hairs on my arms stood straight up as my body savored every second of the sun's magical warmth. My bones felt less achy as the sun warmed them up. Feeling the sun was refreshing.

After the brief moment of enjoyment, we were back to reality: the ride home. This would be the worst part of leaving the hospital. I hadn't sat down normally since the surgery, and sitting in a car hurt unbelievably. It felt like I was sitting on sharp knives because my insides were still very much healing. My stomach was still full of staples and some bandages, and every bump threw my body into a shock wave of pain. This lasted the whole ride home.

Before my surgery, I'd never paid attention to the bouncing around that comes with riding in a car. After the surgery though, I felt every single little bump on the road for that hour and a half car ride home. It was awful, not to mention the road we take home out of Manhattan hasn't been paved probably since the 1800s and is notorious for being in horrible condition.

Not only did we have to go on that road, but it was one of the longer roads that led to the highway. I was in shock and hurting the entire drive home, begging for us to hit Hopatcong so I could finally get out of the car and lay down off of my bottom. When we finally got back into Hopatcong, the battle at Mount Sinai was over; but now it was time to fight the battle in my own home. My hospital trip of eleven days was indeed the worst eleven days of my life to this date, and that will likely stand the test of time. The next couple of weeks at home recovering, however, would give that hospital trip a run for its money.

# CHAPTER 10

# ROCK BOTTOM

———

Health is something we so often take for granted when we're young. I remember being younger and getting birthday cards from loved ones; the cards would have well wishes and in those well wishes was "good health." To me it always sounded corny, and I thought it was something people said that didn't hold much meaning, like small talk.

It's hard to realize how important your health is if you haven't had it in jeopardy. Some things you do every single day seem so normal, so mundane that you don't realize they are gifts—such as getting out of bed, being able to lay in bed comfortably, being able to walk around on your own, eat whatever you want, hang out with your friends, and drive a vehicle. All these things are norms in life you don't think twice about, and you certainly don't correlate them with your health.

Prior to me going through my bout of health issues, I certainly took my health for granted. When I got home from the hospital, I would learn the hard way how valuable and how fragile life is. I was living a second life now, one that was totally different from the life I had previously lived a month ago. That life was dead and gone, buried, forever a part of the past. My new life had a list of obstacles I now had to tackle head on every single day.

In my new life, I couldn't lay down in my own bed when I got home. The staples on my stomach. and the pain my body would be in if I stretched my stomach out was unbearable. In the meantime, I was relocated to the couch where I had to sleep in a reclined position. My abdomen was in so much pain that I was perpetually hunched over. I couldn't stand up straight, lay down, or do anything that stretched my stomach out in the slightest. Aside from not being able to sleep in my own bed, and barely getting five hours of sleep on a nightly basis, my posture began to take a hit. Being constantly bent over when you've lost all your weight doesn't feel good on your back.

My independence was another thing taken from me in my new life. If I wanted to get up and walk around, someone in my family would have to be my personal crutch as I shuffled around the house like a senior citizen. If I wanted to get out of the house, I would have to sit in the passenger seat on a donut so my butt wouldn't be in pain. Everywhere I went, I had to bring a ton of water so I wouldn't dehydrate in the summer sun (I dehydrate quicker now that I don't have a large intestine), and I had to bring a "go bag" with ostomy supplies in them in case I had an emergency.

On a day when I was feeling good, the mental barrier that was enforced on my life was the most difficult thing to get over. If I wanted to see my friends, I would get anxious. *What if they see my bag? What if my bag leaks in front of them? What if I go out in public and it leaks?* The easy short-term conclusion that I came to was I simply wouldn't see my friends or go out in public. I'd be a hermit for the summer, and when this bad dream was over, we could pick my social life back up.

Being couch-locked for weeks after a brutal eleven days in the hospital can take a toll on your mental health. I thought being a hermit would spare me from experiencing more pain, but I couldn't have been more wrong. Maybe that was the outsider talking.

After I had gained some of my strength back, my parents thought this would be a good time to take a nice hot shower for the first time in weeks. It was the one aspect I was looking forward to the most after sitting in my own filth for a week, getting sponge baths from nurses. Little did I know that showering required a great deal of strength—strength I didn't quite have yet.

Showering wasn't the simple daily task for me anymore. Showering had a list of obstacles I had to overcome, much like everything else in my life. The first obstacle was finding the strength to get off the couch and into the bathroom. After that, I had to change my bag before I showered, which was new to me. If I showered with it on, the adhesive would get loose, and you can imagine how that can be a problem. We learned our lesson once before, and the last thing you want is an ostomy leak on your couch because I was too upset to take the bag off while I showered. I began to quickly learn that refusing to care for myself had more negative repercussions than accepting my reality, which would be a pivotal lesson I had to learn on my own.

As I was about to jump into the shower, I looked into the mirror and stared at my own reflection. My face was pale white, with dark circles under my eyes. It looked as if I hadn't slept in days, which was true. My cheeks looked like they were sucked in, with all the weight drained out of my face.

My neck resembled a strip of pencil lead as it connected to my emaciated body. All of my ribs were showing on both sides of my body. Below my ribs was my intestine poking out of my body. Rudolph's nose was emerging from my abdomen. Off center from my intestines was my scar being held together by my staples. The wounds were still fresh with dried blood still occasionally seeping out of the openings. The dried blood acted as glue for the staples as they lay embedded into my flesh. I looked as if I had been liberated from a Nazi concentration camp.

As I analyzed my appearance, I stared in disbelief. I came close to crying, but I was numb at this moment. I still couldn't process this was now the reality of my life. A couple of months before I didn't think I had anything wrong with me. I was a naive teenager, and now I was an adult fighting to come back from the brink. All that time when I was ignorantly running around in childhood bliss, my health was ailing beneath the surface. My genetics were turning against me, and my own body was deteriorating. I just didn't know it yet. A constant reminder of how quick life can change on a dime and that we don't always know what's happening beneath the surface of our own skin.

After I was done being somber over my diminished appearance, I hopped in the shower, hoping it would bring me some relief to at least feel clean. After three minutes, I cut the shower short because I began to feel short of breath. I started to get dizzy, and when I got out of the shower, I told my parents something wasn't right. They told me to go lay down, and when I did, I saw stars. So many stars. My vision was partially blinded for the moment. I fought passing out and laid down, hoping my stamina would be restored soon.

Laying on my bed that night, in my towel, too weak to even get dressed before I almost passed out, was a reminder just how far I was from being "normal"—if I was ever going to be "normal" again. I couldn't stand in a shower for a couple of minutes without losing control of my body. *If I can't shower, then what the hell can I do?*

The one constant throughout my first recovery was the mental battle I was being put through. My faith was questioned repeatedly as I couldn't understand why I was going through this ordeal. I grew up around faith and religion; it wasn't foreign to me. I wouldn't say I wasn't a believer, but to be fair, I never gave it much thought. After coming face to face with my mortality, however, I did start to wonder about faith more and anything beyond this life. It started first with acknowledging all of the horrible things that happen in the world and the suffering we all inevitably go through, even if we are good people.

If God exists, why do people suffer from horrible diseases? Why do good people suffer from unspeakable illnesses? What is the purpose of this life if we are all so damn fragile? How do I find the strength to get through this? Will I be able to get over this? Or was my life doomed to be miserable from a young age?

My energy and will to accomplish the simplest of tasks was also at an all-time low. I wasn't interested in any of the things I used to be. I thought being home would fix feeling this way, like my bed, video games, and being comfortable in my own house. But it didn't; it wasn't the same anymore. When I lost my independence, it felt like my life held very little meaning. It's hard enough to maintain high self-esteem and confidence when everything is going *right*. It feels nearly impossible to fake a smile and act like I'm doing okay when the shit has hit the proverbial fan.

In the hospital, I thought I had hit rock bottom already, and now that I was home, it was time to start climbing out of the pit. I was wrong. My independence was completely stripped from my life and I was now dependent on other people for most things. I didn't know how to adjust to this change in lifestyle. I was still numb from the initial shock of my hospital nightmare.

I would sit on the couch and blankly stare into the TV. My days when I was home were depressing. I would wake up in the morning, after getting an hour of good sleep (if I was lucky) in between tossing and turning in pain all night. There was no movie, no TV show that could make me forget about the pain that hijacked my life. Not even *Breaking Bad* could solve my depressive episodes, and any person who knows me on a personal level knows if *Breaking Bad* can't fix the issue, nothing can. It was going to take some time and *actual effort*—not looking for distractions. Actual effort such as walking around even though it hurt, forcing myself to eat even though my appetite was diminished, and to take care of myself, which meant taking responsibility of my ostomy. That's a key point to remember.

I would pass the time each day by counting down the minutes and the seconds until it was time to go to sleep. Sleep was the only time when I was at ease. I wasn't conscious, so I didn't have a million thoughts persistently running through my head. The pain that consumed my body was gone when I was asleep.

When I was awake, I had to soak in my negativity and process the awful thoughts going on in my head. I couldn't ignore them and push those thoughts to the side for a later time. *I was addicted to the negativity.* I didn't believe there was a light at the end of the tunnel, and I was convinced things would only get worse. I was stuck in the loop of a negative self-fulfilling prophecy.

Every day when nighttime came around, I would spiral out of control. Everyone in my family would be asleep. My mom would be sleeping on the couch adjacent to me in the living room in case something happened in the middle of the night where I needed her assistance. My brother and my dad were usually downstairs, so I would be awake on the couch, scrolling on my phone—scrolling and seeing my friends doing things I would kill to be doing. I would've given up anything at that moment to be able to sleep in my bed, let alone go out with my friends. This is when my mind was at war with itself. I started to feel the distance, the gap, between me and my friends. I was growing apart from my peers whom I knew my entire life. I was so desperate to talk to somebody, to have anybody by my side who would take away even a small piece of the pain. I was *lonely* in these moments. Like I mentioned in Chapter Eight, loneliness kills. When I was in this mood, I would often reach out to people to vent.

Sometimes they would reach back; other times, it would be a while to hear from them. For me, I had nothing going on. I was sitting, waiting for anything good to happen to take my mind from all the pain that had been going on in my life. I spent most nights up until three in the morning not being able to sleep because I could never get comfortable. As I scrolled, I saw friends at a concert that I foolishly thought I would be able to attend; *that hurt to see.* It was painful to see a lot of things that I *should've* been a part of, like graduation parties. Seeing them play out online was definitely a punch in the gut and an aspect my family never had to deal with. This one was unique to me because of my age.

Reaching out to vent was a mistake. The only person who could save me from my demons was me. No other person could magically absorb my pain and make it go away. No amount of kind words that friends could say would help me get better. The only way I could get better was by finding a way to change my own thoughts.

As I started to isolate myself, I held grudges toward people who did not understand my pain, which was definitely not rational. I pinned my problems and anger on others, but the reality was, I was mad at the world. My frustration was bubbling up, and I was reaching a boiling point.

After repeating the same cycle of misery, mixed with sleep deprivation during my first week back home, I became almost catatonic. I don't know how to explain it except to say the pain constantly surrounding me stopped. The mental anguish, the voices in my head saying to give up, and the thoughts of life never getting better were gone. It was like my mind hit the off switch and gave up. I went from over-thinking every waking second to not caring about anything. I reached a scary point in my recovery—one where I felt I had nothing to lose, and I genuinely stopped caring.

I didn't have any interest in having friends come over for visitors. I didn't care to reach out to people anymore, and if they reached out to me, I'd take my time getting back to them. Some people I straight up ignored. I would go to bed not caring if I woke up the following morning. *Why would I want to wake up to relive the same hell all over again?* When my dad, mom, or brother would sit on the couch next to me, trying to cheer me up, I ignored them with the same blank stare of indifference. Reflecting on it now, I would love to go back in time and smack some sense into myself. All I was doing during my self-loathing was hurting those who *actually* loved me the most. I was ripping their hearts out by continuously moping around, and not engaging with anybody. In their defense, my family and friends tried their hardest.

What I was going through was something more common than I realized at the time. I was experiencing post-surgery depression, which according to a 2016 study showed that people who experience chronic pain are more likely to be depressed.[22] Chronic pain is associated with most surgeries, and I sure as hell fit that criteria. It's also noted in that study the combination of surgery, anesthesia, and depression may result in a significant increase in morbidity and mortality for patients.[23]

I will never forget the exact moment when I hit rock bottom. After weeks of my family being patient with me, trying to cheer me up, their patience was running low. They knew I was upset, and they figured this was all normal. After a while of not doing anything to better myself, my mom started to subtly push me along. She would try to get me to run errands with her during the day.

"It's a beautiful day! Come take a ride with me to run a couple of errands? It won't be long, and you don't have to come in," she asked in a peppy voice.

"I don't want to go. I don't feel good," I said bluntly.

"You're never going to feel better being a couch potato. Come on," she demanded.

---

22  Mohamed M Ghoneim, and Michael W O'Hara, "Depression and Post-operative Complications: An Overview," BMC surgery, BioMed Central, February 2, 2016.

23  Ibid.

"I guess I have no choice, huh?"

"Nope, you don't. The sun will feel good. Let's get you some fresh air."

My mom grabbed my tube to sit on for the car seat. I sat on my tube, shamefully, and bounced from location to location with my mom. My mom was trying to make me feel comfortable. She was putting in overtime to put a smile on my face. This is another moment I wish I could go back and slap my stupid, selfish self in the face for breaking my mother's heart.

"You can put your music on if you like. I'll turn off my Bruce." For my mother to offer my music (which she absolutely hated), over her favorite artist, Bruce Springsteen, was her trying absolutely everything for me.

"You don't like my music."

"Yeah…but you do, and I want you to be happy."

"It's alright, I'm not in the mood to listen to music. You can play your Bruce."

It might not seem mean to say, but those words were a knife right into my mom's heart, and it showed on her face. I literally watched my words suck the happiness out of my own mother's face and replaced it with a look of deflated defeat. I saw but didn't care enough to make it right; I was glad she stopped talking to me so I could go back to sulking, staring out the window as she blasted her music. She was blasting her music, but she wasn't singing. Her face had the same disgruntled look on it as mine.

As we rounded back into town, my mom made one last attempt to put a smile on my face.

"Do you want to stop at Fuddruckers for lunch?" my mom asked.

"Yeah, that sounds nice." I was starving, and I loved Fuddruckers. Little did I know this would be another mistake in the recovery process.

My diet had to be monitored, and I essentially had to learn to eat all over again. I had to try small serving sizes of foods to see what agreed with me and what didn't. If something got me sick, we would put it on a list that read "DON'T EAT" hung on the refrigerator. If something didn't give me any problems, we would put it on the "CAN EAT" list.

The list of stuff I couldn't eat looked like a long-form column from the *New York Times*, while the yes list was a few bullet points. Examples of food or drinks I couldn't eat included soda, coffee, any fast food, beef, seafood, any nut, any food with seeds, and most fruits. After I had this realization, my appetite which was on life support as it was, completely evaporated. Eating was now a chore for me, and I had to do it three times a day for my *survival*. I felt like I was completely stripped of my humanity. Eating is something most people can do without thinking about it, and they enjoy it. I was stripped of the enjoyment of food.

The Fuddruckers didn't agree with me and wound up giving me horrendous abdominal pain. I was grimacing in pain for the remainder of the afternoon after briefly enjoying the meal. In a twisted way, this more or less summed up the state of my life at the time: glimpses of simple pleasure, then hours of tortuous pain. Any time it looked like normalcy was being assimilated into my life, it got yanked away from me like I was being taunted. Both of my mother's kind gestures fell flat on their face, and she could sense my sadness deepen.

My dad would try to cheer me up by bringing me home Cliff's milkshakes, which were my favorite from this local ice cream shop by us. That wouldn't help me either; like I said, they tried everything. No one else could snap me out of my funk, but me—I just didn't know this yet. They were trying their hardest though. My dad's frustration began to mount as he wanted to see his son happy again. He wanted me to be with my friends and get back to normal. He didn't understand the fears I had with the bag. The fear of it leaking in public, the fear of it smelling in public. He didn't get it and how could he? It's impossible to explain it unless you lived through it.

What I failed to realize in the moment while I was blinded by my sadness is my parents were battling a plethora of mixed emotions as well. After all, this condition is genetic, so they knew it was a possibility when they decided to have kids. It was a risk, like anything in life, which is why my dad wanted to take the chance. Not to mention we had the worst-case scenario planned out by having a group of great doctors on standby who have been operating on us for four generations. But by me not accepting the reality of my situation and not making an effort to get better, I was making them think maybe it was a mistake to decide to have children. If I had given up, it would wreck them mentally.

I never realized any of these things in the moment. I didn't realize my parents were battling guilt and anxiety like I was. I didn't realize how much my negative emotions were impacting my family and loved ones. I was so selfish, and I could have lived without realizing any of the pain I caused my parents if it wasn't for what happened next.

My mom and I had a heart-to-heart conversation one day when I was on the couch. She tried getting through to me by asking me what was on my mind.

"Come on, sweetie. Can you please let me in? Tell me what you're thinking, please. Even if it's bad, you can talk to me," my mom begged.

"Well, you want to hear what's been on my mind?" I asked curiously.

"Yes, that's what I want. You can tell me anything. I know how tough this is. You can be honest with me. We love you, and we are concerned for you."

I contemplated for a few moments while I sorted through my feelings.

"If you want me to be honest with you, well, the truth is, if I knew this was going to happen to me…I wish I would have never been born at all."

Even writing that memory out onto paper pulls on my heart strings. I still shed tears when I think about how cold, heartless, and mean this moment was. The funny part is, I never intended for it to be mean and heartless. I thought I was such a burden at the moment, that those words wouldn't hurt my mom. I thought it would liberate her to hear that. *What on Earth was I thinking…*

After I uttered those disgusting words, they echoed in the hollow silence that was my living room. My mom's face turned pale white, and she didn't say a word. She took a step back, and the conversation died as quickly as it started. She walked out of the living room and sat on the deck by herself. I sat in the living room continuing the ritual of being miserable on the couch.

My dad came home from work shortly after, and he immediately sensed something was wrong.

"Where's your mother?" he asked, concerned.

"She's on the deck."

He went to the deck to check on my mom. He was out there for about ten minutes, and when he came back into the living room, his face was full of anger. It wasn't seething anger; rather, it was disappointing anger, and most of all it was genuine concern.

"Did you tell your mother you wished you were never born?" he asked me with a disgusted expression on his face.

"She asked me how I felt," I shot back blankly.

"Do you know she is crying on the deck right now? Do you know she is blaming herself right now?"

My heart dropped at the sound of my mom crying and me realizing that it was pretty much all my fault. I was such a fool; I was so blinded by my own sadness. I was so depressed that I hadn't thought about the severity of my words. That was the truth at that moment; that was how I felt. My mom thought that was me confessing I hate her; what my mom heard was, "I have this, and it's all your fault my life sucks."

She thought she was a bad parent and a bad person for this. It breaks my heart even more because during this period of time, I loved my family, and I didn't want them to be so sad anymore. Little did I know on this day I ripped their hearts out and spat on it. The guilt I felt knowing I caused this mess ate at me. I had to make it right, but the question became how?

For the first time in a while, I was looking for solutions even if I didn't necessarily have them, which was a huge step for me considering I wasn't trying prior to this moment. It was almost instinctual. All my self-loathing, the nothingness going on in my head, was gone. All of sudden I snapped back into focus, and the clouds blocking my brain were gone. It was like light was allowed into the shadowy abyss of my consciousness.

"Why is she so upset? This isn't her fault," I sheepishly said to my dad.

"Are you kidding me? She has been feeling like this since you were diagnosed long before your surgery. She doesn't show it. I know this is tough, and we're not saying this is going to be easy. But you need to do this for your mother's sake because if you don't get over this, she isn't going to get over this."

This was a damn shame because my mom explained this to me in the hospital. I let it slip my mind and still believed the delusion from the outsider that I was a burden that needed to be ridded of for my family to ever obtain any normalcy.

He walked back outside to console her, and I sat there replaying what happened over and over—just like the hospital memories, replaying. I didn't want to sit their basking in that moment, but my mind kept running it back on a loop, except this time, the reanalyzing of this situation in my mind helped me in the long run. Much like the hospital memories, I didn't want to relive this trauma. But because I was reliving it, I knew I had to make things right moving forward. The severity of the situation dawned on me from all that analyzing. The severity being, *if I don't pull it together, I might destroy my family!*

The memory of my dad talking to me, saying how he was disappointed in me, and hearing my mom sob in the background knowing it was all *my* fault was devastating for me. It was a turning point; I didn't hit rock bottom. I slammed into it, flipped over a couple times, and then stopped. It was time to pull myself out of the ashes and get my act together. If not, the ramifications of my choices could hurt my family and those who love me.

# CHAPTER 11

# THE CLIMB BACK

---

In the aftermath of my encounter with rock bottom, I had to begin the long ascent back to the top. The first step to making things right had to be the biggest attitude adjustment of my life. I had to apologize to my family for hurting them and being so inconsiderate. I took my dad's advice of making things right with my mom. A couple of hours had passed while I was reflecting on what I had said and my mother's reaction. After a while I decided to confront the moment head on sooner rather than later.

"Hey Ma," I said in a soft voice as I peered into her room, "can I come in?"

She sat on the bed, wiped her eyes, and nodded her head. She had clearly been crying.

I took a couple steps into the room. "I wanted to say that I didn't mean what I said and I'm sorry." I paused and shook my head, fighting emotions of shame. "This is difficult and not easy, but I don't put any blame on you. I don't want you to feel that way."

My mom sat on the bed listening, nodding a little bit. "It's not easy to not blame yourself when you know, logically, this happened because of you."

I interrupted her, "This is no one's fault. Stop it. Especially not yours."

"You swear?"

"I swear." I wiped a tear from my eye. "I had a moment, but I'm going to get better. We're going to get through this. Can we please move forward? I feel terrible about this."

My mom smiled slightly. "Obviously we can move forward. I love you more than anything in the world." I walked over to her bed, and we hugged. Some tears from both of us streamed down our faces. It was difficult—perhaps the most difficult moment in my young life to right this massive wrong I had made.

After the apology, it was time to put my money where my mouth was. I had to show I was doing better, to alleviate the stress on their minds. If I wasn't feeling particularly peachy, they wouldn't know because I would deal with it in private.

My meltdowns and fits of wondering what life would be like did not magically disappear. I feel it is important to clarify to anyone who is reading this and is suffering through a dreadful stretch of events. It isn't a switch you can flip on and off. I would deal with them early in the morning when everyone was sleeping or at night when the day had ended. By myself in my room, I would let my emotions funnel out of me. Sometimes I would vent to a friend if I was having a particularly rough day.

Luckily for me, I had the best support system to build me up from my lowest moment. My family wasn't upset with me and totally understood where I was coming from. I still felt guilty for putting them through so much, and this was something I wrestled with for a while. When it would consume my thoughts, I would remind myself it wasn't my fault; I'm ill right now. I wasn't going to blame myself or add on to beating myself up. I already had enough on my conscience. I didn't need to be my own worst enemy.

Besides, I came up with a way to compensate for this guilt, and that helped. My compensation method was to be emotionally present with my family. I would engage in conversations with them, and I wouldn't be cold toward them anymore. I would make active efforts to tell them how much I appreciate them and to be a rock for them.

The next step on the road to recovery was something I wrestled with quite a bit. It was probably the main reason for the mental slump I was in. It was confronting the ostomy and taking care of myself. The reality was, I needed to live with it for the next three months regardless of how much I despised it. It wasn't going to magically disappear if I kept wishing it away. There was nothing to undo what was already done. I comforted myself with the thought that this won't be my reality for the rest of my life. This will only be my reality for three months. And these three months are going to be an absolute drag if I live as a hermit refusing to take care of myself. If I wanted to take some stress off my family, I was going to have to manage the ostomy on my own with no help. I had to show I can be independent again.

We started with baby steps, such as figuring out how to change it myself. Then, the next step was determining the best time of day to change it, which turned out to be after I showered early in the day when my stomach was empty. I had to play around and fiddle with it, but eventually, I had a system for it. I couldn't do much physical activity during my stretch with the ostomy and standing on my feet for a couple minutes would totally gas me. Building back my stamina was arduous, and throughout my three months of recovery it only slightly improved, so that was a constant battle. Next was to figure out what foods agreed with me and which foods didn't. Any food with nuts or seeds was off limits for me because they don't get fully digested in the small intestine, and that could lead to a blockage. If there is anything worse than an ostomy, it's having a blockage.

Once I confronted the issue of taking care of the ostomy and putting on a strong face for my family moving forward, I had to begin the acceptance process. I had to process and accept that I had my ostomy and to be honest about it. I had visitors dropping by, family and friends, to check on me during this time. I knew at some point I would have to tell them about the second surgery and that I have an ostomy. Part of me debated on if I wanted to mention it or not, considering it was going to be gone in three months. I could have easily made the choice to not talk about it with people outside of my immediate family. I could have distanced myself from people, kept it quiet, and then returned to my social life after I got reconnected.

But then I began to think to myself, *Am I being a fraud?* I'm not open and accepting of my reality if I'm hiding it from people, especially people who say they love and care about me. If they love and care about me, they will accept me for who I am, and realize this isn't my choosing to have this. It doesn't make me less of a person because I have this situation. Anyone with an ounce of compassion can realize these things, and anyone who couldn't realize this, then to hell with them. *Who needs people in your life who look down on you or judge you because of a medical condition?*

If anything, this would be a test to show me who was phony and who was actually there for me. Granted, I was a bit nervous to see the results of this test because I was afraid of losing some people close to me or having people gossip about what happened to me if I opened up. After spending the first couple weeks wrestling with this dilemma, I decided to make a choice to not be a fraud to myself.

So, I opened up, and much to my surprise, I was met with pretty much unanimous support. Some of my friends were upset I had to live through it and were concerned about my well-being. Once I assured them I was going to be fine and this is temporary, no one had a problem with it. Some of my friends and family thought it was cool and couldn't believe that when the beige bag unclipped and the adhesive was removed, that my intestine was on the outside of my body.

I'm sure some people heard rumors through the grapevine about what happened to me, and perhaps they gossiped about me. Perhaps they joked about me, who knows. All I know is anyone who pokes fun at someone based on appearances or based off an illness, it says more about them than it does about me.

Once I let my skeletons out of the closet and had no secrets to hide, I became liberated in a sense. I didn't have to worry about what would happen in public if the bag leaked, or if there was an accident, or if there was an episode around friends and family. That no longer mattered because there wasn't anything to hide and they understood. Some people even admired that I was being open about it. Admiration was never something I thought I would receive before I began to make amends for the wrongs in my life.

---

The rest of the summer, and the months leading up to my second surgery, were still very different. Mentally I made an adjustment that pushed me in the right direction, but physically, I was still reeling. The first month I was pretty much couch-ridden, and everyone visited me at my home if they were to see me. I still needed help walking around the house. I still couldn't lay on my back. I still had staples in my stomach holding me together, and my wound still looked raw and fresh. Standing on my feet for short periods of time hurt me. Almost anything would cause me pain.

After my mom had used her sick days up watching me at home, she would bring me to my grandma's where she would take care of me. My grandma wouldn't be working and always loved having a grandchild over for a visit. She knew what I was going through, so she insisted I come by since I still couldn't be on my own.

These visits at my grandma's were some of my favorite memories from that summer. I would get there early in the morning and we'd have breakfast. She would cook eggs for me and let me eat on the couch where we would watch television. The TV would essentially be background noise as me and my grandma would start talking on a deeper level. She knew I had a lot on my mind, but she didn't force me to talk. She would allow me to talk about what I was comfortable with. At first it would be about trivial things such as sports or movies and what not. Then it would evolve into the elephant in the room, which was me recovering from this condition.

At first, my grandma would tell me stories about when she went through her health battle. She would sit propped on the couch, in her furry bathrobe with long sleeved pajamas on underneath because she was always cold. Her short hair stopped symmetrically at shoulders length. Glasses clung to her nose.

"You know Michael, me and your Aunt Ronnie were quite the guinea pigs back in the day," she interjected.

I cocked my head and squinted. I was a bit confused. "Guinea pigs?"

"Yes, medical guinea pigs. They didn't know me or Ronnie had it at first."

I looked at her with a perplexed expression. "How did you find out?"

Gram shifted in her seat indicating she was about to drop a bombshell on me. "Well, my mom passed suddenly when we were both young. They didn't know what killed her, until they later found out her colon perforated. After that happened, they found out she had FAP. Back in the day, they didn't know if it was genetic, but it was an assumption. So, that's when we got tested afterward."

I sat back looking at her, walking in her shoes in my imagination for a brief second. She was seventeen years old when she lost her mother suddenly, whom she loved very much. My grandma wasn't close with her dad, and from what I've heard, he wasn't a good man. My grandma didn't mention him much, and I didn't prod. The point being, she lost the one parental figure in her life that she loved. That is traumatic and devastating alone for someone to go through. Then imagine my grandma being told she and her sister might have the condition that killed their own mother? I couldn't imagine being in her shoes, yet here she is sitting across from me telling me this story with a mug of tea in her hand.

"Wow...That must've been tough, Gram."

She shrugged her shoulders. "It was tough, but what choice did we have, you know? I'm blessed to have such good people around me who love me. God has been good to me."

My grandma thanking God made me realize why she was probably so spiritual and religious. She probably adopted religion to deal with all the stress and trauma she endured as a kid. It gave her strength; it began to click a little more for me.

"I'm lucky I had your grandfather to be there by my side through it all. Lord knows what I would've done without him. He was my rock."

I shook my head as it made sense, perhaps more sense now than before. I always knew my grandparents loved each other, and that they had a special love story. Married for sixty years and having grown up across the street from each other, they were soulmates. They had the love story from a 1950s black-and-white romantic movie, the type of love stories that don't exist anymore or rarely do. My grandma always emphatically exclaimed how they were soulmates to us all the time. I never doubted them, but I saw the *meaning* behind their relationship. They were kids when their lives were turned upside down. Poppy was the rock for my grandma after losing her mother and to guide her through her health issues. They weren't just a couple; they were life partners on an adventure that had its fair share of bad moments. Their perseverance through those bad moments is why their love was so strong. It's also why *they* were both so strong. Anyone who met them knew how kindhearted and sweet they were, and you'd never believe the obstacles they overcame in their lives.

"So, what happened after that, Gram?"

"Well, Ronnie was diagnosed and had to get her large intestine removed. I wasn't diagnosed until I started showing symptoms, and I was sick when they operated on me. They couldn't remove the rectum back in the day, and they connected our small intestine to the rectum in the meantime."

"So, if they couldn't remove it and they left it, then what?"

My grandma laughed a little bit. "Good question, Michael. You'll never believe it."

I looked at her waiting for further explanation.

"They had to burn the polyps out of our rectums. The only other option was getting a bag, but your Aunt Ronnie and I didn't want that—not initially, so we figured we would burn the polyps out until they couldn't anymore."

I interrupted her momentarily. "How long did you do that for?"

"Oh, about two years I believe," she said casually. "Sure enough, after a while they had to stop because if they continued it would run the risk of the rectum perforating. Plus, the polyps weren't going away either."

"So what happened next?" I sat on the edge of my seat listening to every word of her wild medical stories.

"Well, that's when we went to an ostomy meeting in Livingston. Me and your Aunt Ronnie wanted to see what our reality was going to be. But we got lucky at this meeting."

My grandma wasn't lying when she said she got lucky. They couldn't use names, but someone at the meeting mentioned a doctor in New York who was working on a groundbreaking procedure overseas with a Swedish doctor. Aunt Ronnie's husband, my Uncle Jack, worked in the city and worked on flagging down any information about this miracle working doctor. Sure enough he found him, and his name was Dr. Gelernt.

Dr. Gelernt was a world-renowned surgeon at the time. He became famous for his ability to perform an internal reservoir for patients who suffered from bowel diseases, eliminating the need for an ostomy.[24] This was unheard of during the time period. The procedure was called a Kock Pouch. Dr. Gelernt had traveled to Sweden in 1970 to learn the procedure from the creator himself, Dr. Nils Kock.[25] Dr. Gelernt and Dr. Isadore Kreel was the first to perform the surgery in the United States at Mount Sinai Hospital.[26] My grandma and my Aunt Ronnie were told they were the thirteenth and fourteenth in the world to get the Kock Pouch procedure. My grandma was positive they were the first two to get it in the United States. I couldn't confirm that information.

The procedure from my understanding of how my grandma explained it to me is she had an internal reservoir with a valve that would open when a tube was inserted into her stoma.[27] The stoma I had with my ostomy was visible on the outside of me. My grandma had a tiny hole that could be covered up with a Band-Aid or gauze, and when she went to the bathroom, she had to insert a tube into the reservoir. This way, no bag is needed to be attached to your waist; you just have to insert a tube. This might sound completely outdated but for this time period it was absolutely groundbreaking stuff. This is what exploded Dr. Gelernt onto the scene of the medical industry. It restored some independence to patients

24  Wolfgang Saxon, "Irwin M. Gelernt, 60, Surgeon Specializing in Intestinal Disease," The New York Times, July 4, 1996.

25  Don Schiller, The Kock Pouch procedure (Koch Pouch) and other Ileostomy options - KockPouch.com, 2009.

26  Wolfgang Saxon, "Irwin M. Gelernt, 60, Surgeon Specializing in Intestinal Disease," The New York Times, July 4, 1996.

27  Don Schiller, The Kock Pouch procedure (Koch Pouch) and other Ileostomy options - KockPouch.com, 2009.

who were insecure about having an external reservoir and the issues associated with it.

As my grandma was telling me all these things, I was in awe. I couldn't understand how my petite grandma, who never acted her age a day in her life, endured all of this suffering. Not only endured it but came out on the other side of it so gracefully. Not to minimize what I was going through, but in comparison to my grandma, it was a cakewalk for me. My grandma had to live through the uncertainty of if the surgery would work. She faced more uncertainties and adversities than me, that was for damn sure.

After hearing her tell me these wild stories that far outweighed my struggles, I couldn't just give up. These stories reassured me things would get better, and that I can do this. If she can do what she did and not give up, then neither could I—especially since she thought so highly of me and was convinced I was the stronger one, which I do not agree with at all!

At one of my morning visits, my grandma told me a special recounting about my "birth story," as she called it. My mom was told she couldn't have a second child after her surgeries and her first pregnancy. My mom and dad wanted a sibling for my brother, but the doctors insisted it would take a miracle. That was their words: *a miracle.*

After months of trying and not succeeding, my parents thought it wasn't going to happen. They were sad and disappointed until one day when my mom began to feel the effects of pregnancy. She was certain it couldn't be true because of what her doctors told her. She went to get checked, and she was indeed pregnant with me. My parents were elated; they spread the joyful news quickly through my family. My grandma told me she would never forget the day she got that phone call. She said it was a gift from God after all they had been told.

Then, I was born a couple weeks early, on Christmas Eve no less. I was supposed to be born in January after the New Year, but instead I was born on the eve of our Lord, as my grandma put it. She was convinced I was sent here for a reason by God, but we weren't sure of that reason yet. But she was stern there was a reason, and I had to be here to figure that out.

Hearing her stories, sharing that bond of having the same condition, but at the same time hearing about how much more dire her circumstances were gave me fresh perspective. Maybe things aren't as damned as they seem, and maybe one day things could get better. My situation still wasn't ideal, but my circumstances were certainly better than my grandma's. But she did it, and look at her now. She got through circumstances I couldn't fathom, and she was rewarded for it. She was paid in full, happy and healthy with a loving family. Six grandchildren whom she played intricate roles in all of their lives. Both her and my grandpa were there for every graduation, every big game, and gave a loving phone call if they couldn't be there to celebrate in person. They traveled and crossed off things on their bucket list such as going to Alcatraz and Paradise Island in the Bahamas. Even the simple Wildwood family vacations meant the world to them. Their perseverance got rewarded with a life full of meaning and love.

The "birth story" for me solidified it. I wasn't much into faith at this point in my life, but my grandma was all about faith. Faith gave her the strength and reason to endure all those operations. To overcome losing her mother at a young age and the countless other things she rose above. From a logistical standpoint, I understood why my grandma was into faith and religion. I was starting to dabble in it a bit myself now. What this story and spending time with my grandma showed me was that she *believed* in this. I mean she believed in such a way I was able to feel it. Not only was I able to feel it, but I began to reflect on it. *Was it fate that led them to that stranger who recommended them to Dr. Gelernt? Was it fate that my grandma met my grandpa? Was it fate that I was born despite all the odds? Was it fate that I was born on Christmas Eve?*

It was comforting and reassuring; the energy she carried had rubbed off on me. This belief my grandma held became an inspiration for me to make a rapid recovery and turn this into a positive even if it didn't feel like it yet. I was climbing my up from rock bottom.

# CHAPTER 12

# THE LITTLE THINGS COUNT

———

My visits with my grandma helped me to change my attitude on the situation, which was slowly starting to happen. It wasn't a one-night overhaul, where I woke up with smiles and enthusiasm. But I wasn't couch-locked waiting for the sweet release of drifting off into a deep sleep where my mind was no longer harassing me. In other words, I wasn't waiting to die anymore. I was taking initiative to make my life better.

Now that the cat was out of the bag, my friends were aware of what was happening to me. I wasn't running around in public lifting my shirt up to anyone and everyone letting them know about my situation, but I also wasn't hiding what was going on from the people closest to me. I was beginning to do my best job at eliminating the distance I purposely put between me and everyone in my life.

Cleaning up the scraps and debris from those fractured relationships was difficult. It had been effortless to push myself away from everyone during my depressive episode, however. Some people as you might imagine, took me pushing them away quite personally. Others were off put by my attitude in general. With those who weren't off put, I found it difficult to try and fight past the guilt I had of driving this wedge in the first place. I would ignore it and push through it, but it was this nagging feeling that weighed heavily on my mind as I mended the bridges I burned.

This would also be a key theme and lesson I learned during these periods in my life. What I began to notice was there was a necessary process with growth. Anytime I experienced growth in my life, I had to force myself through uncomfortable situations. Situations like mending fractured relationships, taking responsibility of my health condition and my ostomy, getting into physical fitness after all my body has been through, writing a book, and being completely transparent with my struggles. All of these things hurt either mentally, or physically, in the beginning. They made me uncomfortable, but by pushing through the pain I eventually got to a point where there was none. As a matter of fact, things got...better. Doing necessary and meaningful things come with a temporary price of discomfort, followed by a reward of meaning and purpose.

As the summer continued on, the bond I formed with my grandma, my aunt, and my mom molded into something special for all of us. My family as a whole supported me in ways I can never begin to repay. I have a huge Italian family; think of the scene in *Goodfellas* where Karen was saying how there were so many people and all of them were named Peter or Paul, but substitute those names with Anthony. Each member of my family played a vital role in helping me recover, and their acceptance of my situation helped get me on the right path. Having a big family is especially nice when you are close with them.

They know how much they mean to me, and I've told them countless times how much I appreciate their love and support. But the bond between my aunt, grandma, and mom was different because we were the four living with this illness. We are thankful that it is just *us*. It is not something we would wish on our worst enemy, but at times it can get a little lonely, scary, and mentally exhausting to deal with this, with no one to vent to who *has* it. If I was having stomach issues for a week, I would wonder, *Was it something I ate that did it? Do I need to go to the doctor?* Thankfully, I could call my aunt or my grandma really quick and confirm if it was a cause for concern. That is the benefit of having family members who know what you are going through. If we didn't share the same operation, it was a support group. What better support group could you ask for when you already have unconditional love and support from your family?

As the summer progressed, I began to get better. The staples had been taken out of my stomach, so that began to heal. It was no longer a bloody line that looked like it might begin to peel apart if the staples weren't in my skin. I could sleep in my bed, albeit it hurt like hell most nights; it still felt better than being a slave to my living room couch. And by the grace of God, I could shower without almost passing out. Hallelujah.

I could walk around the house without my dad, brother, and mother being my personal set of crutches. I was able to shuffle around the house, although my posture wasn't particularly sexy. I was hunched over as my stomach was still tender and had to be handled with care. So, needless to say I wasn't going to be lifting weights, running marathons, or shooting hoops. But I also wasn't a totally dependent person. That was a nice feeling.

It was also liberating to be able to drive for the first time in months. I didn't have to sit on a rectal donut out in public to protect myself from the excruciating pain of sitting on a hard surface with my boney little behind. My ass was still boney, and it didn't feel the best, but it also didn't cause me to wince in agony anymore. Just a little pain, or maybe it would be painful to someone else. Maybe I adjusted to living in pain, who knows.

I got to the point where the bag wouldn't gross me out. I could change it and look at it without cringing, flinching, or cursing at God for giving me this albatross. Maybe it was because I knew in my mind this was all temporary. Probably. But who cares? After all, that was my situation. If things were different and this was permanent, perhaps I would've still been reeling mentally. It's hard to tell, but I do sympathize with people who live with stomas. And I sure as hell admire the ones that live openly with it and proudly.

Something also began to happen to me as I experienced these "firsts" again. The first time I left the house to go pick up a cup of coffee. This is something I would do, and most of us do, mundanely in our everyday lives. We jump in the car in a rush, speed to our destination taking everything for granted in between. It's not our faults per se, we don't know what it's like to not be able to take a quick drive to Dunkin'; it doesn't pass your mind twice if you're healthy and everything is in order.

Coffee is one of my favorite things ever, and to have it back in my life was a comforting feeling that things would be alright. All it took was getting one of the things I enjoyed so much back into my life to change my perspective. July 10 is when my life as I knew it was derailed. By the beginning of September, with my second operation creeping around the corner, I was able to have this simple joy again for a brief moment in time. It would only be a couple weeks before I was hospitalized again, but damn did it feel good to put the key into the ignition.

I was working at a coffee shop in my town during my high school years. My senior year when I got the news I was going to be operated on, I had to obviously tell my work. When I called the owner of the shop that I worked at, she understood the severity of my situation and told me to take as long as I needed. That I would come back to a job whenever I was healthy again, and of course she wished me well. She was a very kind Irish woman, and I had been working there for three years so we were well acquainted. My manager and co-workers wished me well and we're very supportive. They even sent me get well cards, which they all signed, as I recouped at home. I was concerned prior to getting operated on that I would lose my job, but fortunately, that wasn't the case.

The last time my co-workers and the regulars at my job saw me I was a different person then who I was now. I was transitioning from the first Mike phase of my life, to the second. The second Mike was very slim and frail, it looked like if you pushed him hard enough, he'd tumble backward and break something. He was pale with a thin pencil neck and a poor attempt at a beard. Despite his diminished appearance, he didn't seem discouraged or even bothered. A newfound appreciation became visible from his guarded self prior. Despite his physical ailments, a part of him looked liberated. He certainly didn't look like he was suffering, so that wiped the worry away from his peers and loved ones.

I had pulled into the parking lot for the first time since I got operated on. My style these days wasn't the best, and I mostly wore clothes that were comfortable, especially around my waistline. On that particular day I was wearing basketball shorts, long black socks, flip flops, and a black T-shirt. I hopped out of my car and strolled in to order my first cup of coffee since that dreaded day at the hospital. This time, I knew the end result would be satisfying and not mortifying.

As I walked in, I saw my co-worker and friend Dan working behind the counter. He saw me walk in and flashed me a big smile, followed by, "Look who's back!"

I waved. "Yup, I'm back."

"Are you coming back to work?" he asked, as he examined my physical condition. "You look...."

"Like shit, I know." I finished the thought for him.

"I was going to say thin, but how are you feeling?"

"Actually, not that bad." I smiled. "I think I can work again. Not like I used to, but I want to have some normalcy again."

"Justine is in the back if you want to figure that out with her."

I began to walk behind the counter, "Yeah, while I'm at it, I'm going to make my own cup—gotta make sure it's perfect." I nudged him in a joking matter.

"Oh, so I don't make it good enough?"

I began turning the corner to the office and shot one last look his way. "No one makes it quite like me." He shook his head and smiled as I left the frame.

When I talked with my boss, I explained to her that seven-hour shifts were a thing of the past until further notice, but that wasn't a problem. She could tell with her eyes that I wasn't in the condition to be working for long periods of time. So, we compromised to working three days a week, for three to four hours at a time per week. If I was feeling strong enough, I was always welcome to pick up shifts, no one would ever stop me from doing that if I wanted to. I voiced my concern for the dress code, as wearing jeans was very uncomfortable around my waist, and again, to my surprise, that wasn't a worry. I was able to wear shorts or pants that were a bit more forgiving on the waist as long as they looked like jeans. The beautiful invention of joggers became the primary weapon in my closet arsenal.

All my demands had been met, so I left that day with no concerns. I wasn't bothered by my co-workers noticing my appearance was diminished; anyone with a pair of eyes could see that. It didn't make them a bad person for stating the painfully obvious. It's only natural that people would notice and react in a variety of different ways. It wasn't in a malicious way, so I was able to overlook it.

I left with my perfect cup of coffee and picked up my check. The best part about this trip was the first time I put my lips up to that warm cup. Smelling the aroma of hot hazelnut for the first time made my dopamine receptors happy. They practically climaxed when I was able to gulp down the first mouthful of the creamy substance.

It was the first time since the surgery my taste buds were greeted with the pleasurable taste of coffee. The last time I had coffee was when I had my puking fit in the hospital. Coffee didn't agree with me for the first couple months of my recovery. And, if I were being honest, I was scared to try it after that horrible episode. I wasn't even sure if I could have coffee ever again. I hadn't tried it since my body was working in normal function, and things were different now.

This is exactly why this day was so significant to me. I was starting to see that little glimmer at the end of the tunnel. When I realized I was able to drive again, after having that aspect of my life stripped away from me, the light got a little brighter. When I realized that coffee (my favorite thing on this planet) could officially be taken off the "DON'T EAT" list, the light got a little brighter. I realized the list wouldn't be permanent, and my mind permeated in the feeling of crossing off more of those suckers. Suddenly, it was at this moment I began to undergo a massive perspective shift.

It's hard to describe to people who have never had simple liberties taken away from them at the hands of health issues. Moving toward better health, not perfect health, but enough to where you get some freedoms back, even while still dealing with pain, makes all the difference. Being able to drink coffee again might seem like a minute, insignificant detail, but to me it was a sign my world was beginning to change. This time it seemed like for the better.

For the first time in my life, I understood the seemingly cliche saying of, "It's the little things in life that counts." The corny saying you read on the inside of Hallmark cards or that your aunt says at family reunions, but you think she's a bit cheesy. It isn't cheesy; it is the truth.

This perspective shift made me realize that the mask I had been wearing since my rock bottom moment, was officially off. I wasn't faking it anymore; this was genuine enjoyment. Something I hadn't experienced in months if not a whole calendar year. And it came from doing something so simple. Can I imagine the joy I'd feel when I experience things a bit more significant then drinking a cup of coffee?

# PART IV

# THE ROAD TO RECOVERY

# CHAPTER 13

# THE CLUB

---

As my physical and mental well-being began trending in a positive direction for the first time in months, my family took advantage of it. My comfort zone was still with the people closest to me, my family and immediate circle of friends. I would go to social gatherings, but typically didn't stay super long. Being there was a huge step for me. Plus, my friends understood, and most of the time I would offer being the designated driver for them during the summer of 2015. I was hanging out with them while simultaneously being a help to them, which was a nice feeling considering I was the one who everyone was helping all summer. Totally different circumstances but the role reversal was a nice change of pace. It was probably the only time in my life I didn't mind babysitting my drunk friends.

I didn't have any particularly taxing trips that summer. It wasn't as if I was hiking, swimming, or playing volleyball at the beach. Anything out of the normal was a "club trip." Club trips, as my grandma began to affectionately call them, were ways to do fun things for me during this "new normal" summer. Things weren't normal, and we accepted that as a family. The new normal didn't mean we couldn't have some fun and make the most of it. My grandma wanted to give me some fun memories from that summer, so it wasn't only doom and gloom. We planned our first club trip when my grandma, my aunt, and I were sitting down for dinner one night.

"You know, Michael," she said as she impaled her food with her fork, "I think you're starting to get better to the point that maybe you could go out a little bit, have some fun?"

I smirked as I popped open the takeout container's lid and began to dip my boneless wings into ranch dressing.

*Another thing off the list, for those of you wondering.*

"Yeah, I guess we could, and if anything happens it won't be the end of the world considering it'll be the club."

"Oh honey, we'll be prepared if anything goes wrong, and you know we aren't going to care if something were to happen. Besides, we need to have some fun experiences this summer," she said enthusiastically.

I finished chewing my food to avoid talking with a mouth full of barbeque sauce and shredded chicken. "So, any ideas in particular of what we could do?"

My grandma sat back and began to think. I could smell the wood burning as she thought of some fun ideas.

"Hmm." She closed her mouth and gritted her teeth. "We could go to Tavern on the Green with your Aunt Re. We've always wanted to go but never have. Plus, I know how much you love food."

I let out a chuckle. "I do love food, but the question is what kind of food are we talking about?" I said like a sarcastic smart aleck.

My grandma picked up on the sarcasm I was putting down, smiled, leaned forward and said, "Only the best kinds of food. It's a fancy restaurant in the middle of Central Park. We could knock two birds out with one stone."

"Ah, so that means this is going to be an expensive outing?"

"I can afford it. Besides, that's not any of your concern anyways. The offer still stands; do you want to go? We can plan a date for next week. Maybe make a day out of it and do something in the park."

That did sound pretty nice, and having a day out gave me something to be excited about for the first time in a while. I was a little nervous being out in public, away from my designated safe spots which consisted of my house and my grandma's house. But I felt totally comfortable with my aunt and grandma, so I decided to give it a shot. If I were to start feeling ill or God forbid had an accident, I wouldn't want to be with anyone else.

"Sounds like a plan to me," I said with a stupid grin on my face. "Just know I'm going to get the expensive food."

"Honey, you can get whatever you want."

"Since we're going for lunch, we should probably figure out something to do beforehand," I said, opening the door for suggestions.

My grandma leaned back once again in deep thought. "We can go to the Museum of Natural History—that's always fun. Plus, it's been a long time for me; how about you?"

The last time I was at the Museum of Natural History I was too young to understand much of what I was looking at. "Yeah, that sounds good to me."

"Then it's a date. How's next Thursday sound?"

"Sounds good to me," I replied back, genuinely excited about it.

My mom had been debriefed about me and my grandma's little plan for an afternoon trip. My mother agreed, and when the time came, Thursday, August 27, 2015, we made the first annual "club trip," and more importantly, it was my first big day out in about two months. Up until this moment, I had been cocooning in my humble abodes away from society and potentially embarrassing or painful situations. Plus, at this point in my recovery, it was pretty much doctors' orders to start being active, that is if I wanted to get better. It was the same message I was told during my first trip in the hospital.

It was early in the morning when my mom dropped me off at my grandma's before work. It was early enough where dew glistened on the glass, and the early morning chill sent a shiver down my spine. That wouldn't last too much longer as the sun began to rise from its nightly slumber.

"First big day today. Are you excited?" my mother asked with a big smile across her face.

"Yeah I am; I'm also a bit nervous."

"That's fine; you're with grandma and your Aunt Re. Nobody loves you more than them, other than me of course." She smiled; she thought that was clever. "Besides, this is going to be fun. Enjoy yourself!"

"I know, and I will. Gotta start getting better eventually, right?"

She smiled. "That's the attitude, kid."

I got out of the car and was greeted by my grandma who was standing by the door anticipating my arrival. I had my grey, bland shorts that I wore during this time period since much didn't fit me, and it seemed pointless to buy clothes as I wasn't going to be this thin forever. I hoped not. I had a grey Young & Reckless shirt that was the same shade of color as my shorts and my low top vans.

My style during this time period wasn't particularly stellar. I didn't look great; I accepted that. But I did have on my

Apple Watch on my right wrist that my grandma gave me as a surgery gift during my time recovering. I had gotten a ton of surgery gifts from both sides of my family. Amazon gift cards, an Apple Watch, clothes, cards with warm wishes, and, of course, the universal love language: money.

I had my "go bag" as my aunt called it, which carried all my emergency ostomy supplies in case of emergency. It was in a black Nike string strap athletic bag that swung over my shoulders. I was all set to embark on my first post-surgery adventure that didn't include picking up takeout food.

After I hugged and greeted my aunt and grandma, we quickly got ready as we weren't wasting much time since we had a busy day. Not only did we have a busy day, but we remember just how fun the commute is into the city. So, we began our drive and ended up at the parking lot for the Museum of Natural History. After we paid the parking attendant, we received our ticket, and parked accordingly. It was a beautiful day in the city. Eighty degrees, warm enough to feel the vitamin D being absorbed into my body, but not too warm to turn me into a sweaty mess. Cloud covering seemed to kick in when things crept past the point of discomfort, as a natural neutralizer.

We began with the great Alaskan moose and grizzly bear room. I stood in front of the mirror observing the ten-foot-tall behemoth as the prop towered over me. Brown fur covered in dirt and dust, claws sharp enough to rip me to shreds, and a creepy real look in its eyes. If the bear was alive, I'd be terrified; but knowing it was fake, I could take goofy photos with it and pretend to be macho and unafraid.

I made a silly face and put up my fists as if I was challenging the bear, and my aunt snapped a photo.

"That was a good one! Come check it out." I shuffled over to her and grabbed her phone to observe the photo.

"I look thin. I don't like the way I look." My clothes looked like I was swimming in them, and my buzz cut didn't help add any thickness to my frame. It made me look sicker if anything. My grandma sat back seeing that I wasn't particularly thrilled after seeing myself through the camera.

"Hey Michael, stand up on that bench next to the elephants. Take another picture."

"Just to be goofy? Or for what?"

"Well yeah, be goofy, but I have another idea." She scratched her chin, then crossed her arms. "You're going to look back on this, Michael. You're going to look back and see how far you've come one day. This will be your marker."

"How so?"

"Well Dr. Gorfine said you're about halfway through your recovery. So, this is where you are now, halfway through. We still have a long way to go, and you'll be able to use this moment as a visual medium for when things get better."

I stepped up onto the bench, folded my arms, and made a typical bro pose. My confidence was lacking in this picture, but it was taken regardless.

"Don't worry Michael, it isn't going anywhere. This is for you; it'll stay between the club if that's what you want. But I'm telling you, you'll look back on this fondly one day."

My aunt put her phone in her pocketbook. "Gram is right about this one, sweetie. We've all been at this point. I didn't look great at this phase either; matter of fact, we weren't going on trips like this during my recovery. Not this quickly at least. You're knocking my records out of the park like I knew you would."

I smiled a little bit, almost not believing what she was saying. "Really? You didn't at this point?"

"Medicine was much different back then in '87, sweetie. It was good, better than Gram or your mother, but it's always changing. Back when Dr. Gorfine worked on me, I was his first J-pouch operation where he had help from Gelernt. He's done thousands of these pouches since working on me. He's perfected it."

This was true and still remains true to this day. Medicine advances happen so quickly, almost in the blink of an eye. From my aunt's J-pouch in '87 right up until my operation in 2015, so many medical advances were made. They scrap things that don't work and substitute them for better solutions based on research and data, and this is happening every day. There have been advances from 2015 to the time of this book (2021). For example, my mother from September 2019 through March 2020 had to get a reversal from what she had to a J-pouch operation, something we were told could never be done; reversals weren't possible in 2015. And in 2020, they were relatively routine.

After we had that little moment, we continued on with our afternoon. We stopped by the dinosaur exhibit of the museum, and let's be real, if you don't check out the dinosaur exhibit, did you go to the museum? After we took pictures and observed the fossil recreations of these ancient species that once ruled the planet before humans were a thing, we had worked up a bit of an appetite, which meant it was time to hit Tavern on the Green.

"So how are we feeling, Michael? Do we want to continue? Totally up to you don't feel pressured," my grandma said reassuringly, rubbing my shoulders.

"I'm good, we can do it."

"Remember this day is all on how you feel, kiddo. We stop when you stop," my aunt said, adding to the reassuring atmosphere.

"We'll see, but definitely let's get food first."

"That sounds like my grandson!"

We continued to Central Park on this picture-perfect day. Passing by park goers having picnics with family and friends. Some were reading on a blanket, others tanning, some napping right there in the park. People of all shapes and sizes and groups small and large found different ways to take advantage of the beautiful day.

When we finally arrived, we took in the restaurant for the first time. It was huge, and the brick road that greeted you at the front entrance felt like I traveled back in time to the late 1800s. A long red awning paved the way for customers to walk in without getting rained on, if weather conditions were less than favorable. On the front of the awning, the logo of two sheep propping up against a plate that has the name of the restaurant written boldly on it. When we walked down the brick pathway, we were greeted by the host. People were funneling in and out of the restaurant but still there were seats available despite the influx of people.

"Hello, welcome to Tavern on the Green! How many today?" the hostess asked.

"Just us three," said my grandma. She began to point to the left. "Is it possible if we could sit in the glass house area? It's too nice out to be completely inside."

"Sure thing, ma'am. We got spots for you. Follow me."

The host guided us to our seat, and we were in awe of the beauty of the day and restaurant. A glass overhead with a light grey awning let the light in, but not enough to torch us. Behind us was a completely enclosed dining area, and in front of us were clear glass windows that illuminated the entire room. Busy waiters scurried by with cocktails and drinks in their hands rushing to satisfy their tables for a healthy tip. Sounds of people laughing and chatting drowned out any possibilities of an awkward silence.

"Well, if the food sucks at least the place looks awesome," my aunt said, laughing while taking in the atmosphere.

I was rotating my head looking up and down, right to left. "You got that right. This place is bougie."

My grandma laughed. "Yeah Michael, we don't mess around. That's for sure." My grandma reached into her pocketbook, took out her phone, and began taking pictures. "Hey, I don't know when or if I'm going to be here again. My memory isn't the best—let's face it, I'm old, so pictures do what my memory should be doing."

Me and my aunt laughed and looked at each other. She shook her head. "No one was accusing you of that, Mom. Snap away...Actually, I think I'll join you."

"Me too," I said, laughing as I grabbed my phone to capture the moment as well.

We ordered our food, which was absolutely delicious. I had Manhattan clam chowder, because, I mean, we're in Manhattan after all. *This has to be the best authentic Manhattan clam chowder,* I thought to myself. And it was; it blew canned soups and diner knockoffs out of the water. It was also a bit spicy, which opened up my sinuses. My grandma and aunt got the cream of corn soup, which was delicious and better than my soup. I stole some of theirs, and I acted as the human dumpster at the dinner table. Whatever they didn't eat, I did. It was a pretty solid deal if you ask me.

*Check.*

After we ate, I began to feel a bit fatigued. I was tired and a little sore from walking around all day. My stoma had been relatively dormant all morning and early afternoon since I didn't eat much to play it safe. After I ate, my stoma was like Mt. St. Helens, and I could feel it pulsating. This meant that I was going to the bathroom, which made me a bit nervous. This partially contributed to me wanting to wrap the day up. We waited at our table for a bit so that I could go to the bathroom comfortably.

After I went, my grandma asked what the verdict was. "So, how are we feeling? Done or not done?"

I adjusted my belt, winced a little bit, "Well, I'm having a good time, and we're already here. It's just I'm a little tired. I wouldn't mind going through Central Park a bit more, but walking is kind of tough for me right now."

My grandma stood there for a second thinking. I watched her eyes wandering beyond me looking for something.

"A-ha! I got an idea! It'll be my treat too. Let's take a horse carriage ride through Central Park! I've always wanted to do it; I can cross that off my bucket list. We can go to the *Friends* fountain!" My grandma lit up like a kid who was just told they can have whatever they want at the candy shop.

"Are you sure this is for him or for you?" my aunt asked, laughing so hard she could barely get the words out.

"Oh, shut up. It's for him, but I'm allowed to have some fun too."

My grandma was a pip, and when she wanted to have fun, she made it hard to say no. So, I agreed, as I didn't want to stop the afternoon from ending. After all, I hadn't done anything remotely close to this fun and normal since my surgery. I didn't think this would be possible or we would get this far feeling as good as I did, so I definitely wanted to keep the good times rolling.

My grandma flagged down a kind gentleman in a horse carriage to give us a ride through the park. He took us all over Central Park, pointing out famous landmarks and giving the backstory on them to us.

"Special occasion for you guys or what?" asked the tour guide curiously.

"Today is a special day for a special person," my grandma said enthusiastically.

My aunt interjected, finishing what my grandma started. "My nephew, her grandson, right here, is celebrating his half-way point in his recovery from an operation he had about two months ago. Today is a happy day."

"How beautiful of an occasion. I'm glad to hear you're doing well, buddy. Care if I ask what the surgery was?" the tour guide asked as he guided his trusty steed in the right direction.

"It was a big one. You'll never guess it or believe it for that matter," my grandma said with a bit of pride in her voice.

"Try me!"

"Well, we all have the same condition. It's genetic. He had to get his large intestine removed to put it shortly; we all had to do it at one point. We had to do it because without it, cancer grows in our large intestine to put it in simple terms."

The tour guide's eyes widened. His jaw dropped a bit and he said, "Your whole large intestine? Like you don't have any of it? None of you?"

"Nope, all three of us are without it. We are the club," said my aunt laughing.

"Wow…I would've never guessed," our guide said in awe.

"Told you so," my grandma interjected with a smirk.

"Well, God bless you guys; you look good all things considered. And you seem to have the right attitude. You also seem to be close; family is important. It seems like it means a lot to you guys."

"It most certainly does," I said, nodding my head in agreement.

After seeing the tour guide's face, I could tell how lucky I was. My grandma and my aunt spoiled me this entire day just to lift my spirits and show me things will go back to normal. I mean, I told my aunt and my grandma I was tired but still contemplated continuing the day, and what do they do? They treat me to a horse carriage tour through Central Park out of unconditional love.

I sat in the carriage taking in the sights, listening to my grandma and my aunt proudly yap away to the tour guide about our family history and how great I am (it was good for the ego). I stared off into the distance taking in the sights, blissfully smiling as I was appreciating all they had done for me that day. I was appreciating the first good day in a while.

We stopped at the *Friends* fountain, where my grandma was itching to go. She propped up out of her seat, cupped her eyes to see better and began to shout, "There it is! There it is!" My grandma loved the show *Friends*, if you couldn't tell by now.

"Sir, you've been very kind to us," my grandma said to the tour guide. "Would you mind taking a photo of the three of us, so no one is left out?"

"Absolutely, ma'am." All of us disembarked from the carriage and went over to the fountain.

My grandma began dancing and doing silly poses "C'mon, we have to do what they did in the intro! Didn't they have a dance or a pose or something they did? I can't remember."

"I don't remember, Mom. After all, you watch it mostly," my aunt said laughing at Gram being a goofball. Out of the three of us my grandma had the childlike enthusiasm that day.

"Well, let's do something goofy then." She took out her arms and sang the show's theme song. She threw her arm over my shoulder, mine over hers, and my aunt joined in too. All of us were laughing at my grandma's shenanigans.

The tour guide took the photo. "Beautiful!" he said.

My grandma trotted over happily with my aunt to see the photo. "You probably think we're total lunatics."

"Yeah Mom, I think that ship has sailed."

The tour guide laughed as he gave back the phone. "No, no, no, nonsense! You guys are the most entertaining people I've had today. Made my day go by a bit quicker, and a little brighter."

As we proceeded to get back onto the carriage, my grandma spotted a dime on the ground. She bent down to pick it up. I watched her but was confused why she seemed so happy about a dime.

"Why'd you pick up that dime, Gram? Times tough financially?" I joked with her.

She smiled back. "No, Michael. Dimes are a sign from a loved one in heaven. The number ten represents a full circle. It's something I've always believed in."

I smiled at her explanation without further prodding. As I've mentioned before, my grandma was very spiritual, and she had her reasons. I knew she believed, and I didn't want to impede on her sentimental moment. I was still on the fence about things like signs, but that would eventually change over time.

After our tour was done, we wrapped up a long and eventful day full of laughing and having fun. I was exhausted physically, and it did take a toll on my body. But it was totally worth it for a couple of reasons. For starters, it was fun, and I needed some fun memories. It was important for me to have that experience for my mental health. I also needed it for my physical health too, as I needed to start walking around and being out and about. My aunt and my grandma came up with the idea of having another club trip in a couple of weeks, this time with my mom, dad, and grandpa to have an event together as a family, similar to what we did that day since it was such an enjoyable experience for all of us.

# CHAPTER 14

# SURGERY NO. 2

———

As the summer came to a close, I slowly became more self-sufficient, inching my way closer to the anticipated second surgery. Once I started to feel a little better, we were going to be right back at square one in a couple of weeks. One step forward, two steps back.

My family and I did one more club trip with the addition of my mom, dad, and grandpa. We went to the USS Intrepid in New York City, a big old Navy ship with tons of planes and navy equipment on it that my grandpa and dad were gushing over. My dad loves jets, planes, and military stuff. My grandpa was in the Navy, so needless to say, it was exciting for him and he took great pride in explaining to us the intricacies of living on a Naval ship. It was a beautiful September day, sunny with a few clouds in the sky. The Intrepid was indoor and outdoor so we got the best of both worlds. My family did a good job at making that summer feel as normal as it possibly could. I had some great memories that I will hold onto dearly, which is something I never thought I'd say during my time in the hospital.

I followed Dr. Gorfine's instructions to a T. He told me very sternly the things I should and shouldn't be doing. First and foremost was no heavy lifting or vigorous exercise. So, we put the dream of becoming Arnold to the side for the summer—no problems there. The next was developing some strength back through walking and becoming more self-sufficient. We can check that one off the list too, albeit, I was very reluctant in the beginning; I was still able to do those things. I remember Dr. Gorfine telling me that if I followed his rules, there was an outside chance the second surgery could be bumped up a bit. Doing this would mean getting the bag off sooner, which was my dream at the moment.

In early September of 2015, we had our monthly check up with Dr. Gorfine. I'd had one around the end of July to get the staples out and to see how I was doing. I wasn't too sure what this visit would entail since the staples were removed and there was nothing else to take out. Perhaps I could get rewarded with my second surgery being bumped up a couple weeks?

We arrived at Dr. Gorfine's office and got down to business as usual. He felt my stomach and attended to the stoma. He asked me how I was feeling and then began to slap on his latex gloves. "Time to check and see if the pouch is all healed, Michael," he told me as he grabbed some sort of scope.

"Let me guess—this is going to hurt?" I asked, piecing the puzzle together in my head.

He looked at me, shrugged a bit, and said, "Some people say yes, some people say no. It's probably going to be uncomfortable."

I knew the only way he was going to know if the pouch had healed or not was to put that thing where the sun doesn't shine and do some investigating. We don't have to go into the nitty grit as to how this went. It hurt, as you could probably imagine.

"I'll give you a minute if you need it," he said, noticing I was in the demographic of people who would say this hurt. "I'll be in the room with your parents to tell them the news, and it is good news."

After I took a minute to compose myself, I opened the door and walked into his office sitting down gently next to my parents.

"So, Doc, how are things looking? When do you think the next surgery is going to be?" my dad asked.

Dr. Gorfine leaned back in his chair, tapping his pen on the desk as his face was deep in thought. "Things look good; I think he could be ready in two weeks."

My mom and my dad's faces lit up with excitement. "Two weeks, you think?" my mom asked with a big smile on her face.

"Wow, that's great news," my dad said, agreeing with my mom.

Dr. Gorfine continued to look as if he was in deep thought. "I wouldn't schedule without a second opinion, but I can set an appointment for him to get an X-ray to confirm if he's ready."

"You can do that today?" My mom was getting progressively happier.

"Yeah, as a matter a fact, just hold on one second."

Dr. Gorfine made a quick phone call, wrote on a piece of paper the address in the city of the doctor we were going to meet, and told us the doctor would be ready within an hour or so. Just like that I went from routine checkup to being booked early for my second surgery. I was ahead of schedule for once.

My family was super excited as we scurried off to the next address in Manhattan so I could get another series of tests done. Part of me was happy because I was finally going to get this bag off, and I was going to be headed on the road to recovery. It was almost within grasp, and that was exciting. But I was still rattled by the first scope test done back at Dr. Gorfine's office. I was quite embarrassed and in a bit of pain, knowing the pain wasn't going to stop there today. At the same time, I knew that sucking this up would lead to me getting operated on sooner. This was also a mixed bag because I was just as scared to get operated on the second time as I was the first. It is never easy to be put under the knife.

We got to the office and sat in another waiting room decorated in plaques and medical awards. Dr. Gorfine's medical circle was one of the best, and it reflected every time we went to someone under his team. I was called into the back where I had to strip down into a hospital gown. My favorite.

After having my ass exposed to the wind, it was time to go into the examination room. It had white floors and walls with shiny silver equipment everywhere. *Would it kill any of these doctor's offices to have a colorful room that didn't resemble a high school cafeteria?* The view outside the windows wasn't great either, as all I could see were the sides of buildings, with the tiniest sliver of Manhattan skyline. In the middle of the room was a CT scan machine, and it was my first time seeing it. It looked like a big, white letter O that generated a relatively loud humming sound of sorts. It was loud enough to know that the behemoth was producing the noise, but not loud enough to drown out dull conversations. I did not want to be in the middle of that thing as it shoots radiation waves into me, but I did what I was told and got onto the table. When it encompassed my body, I began to feel claustrophobic and anxious, its loud hums taking over my senses.

Little did I know the CT scan was the least of my worries on this day. We went to this doctor's office to see if my J-pouch had healed properly, meaning it wasn't bleeding still, and there were no openings so to speak. This was to make sure that when Dr. Gorfine reconnected my intestines, shit wouldn't be leaking into my bloodstream. There is no way to sugar coat it, that's pretty much what it was for. I'm sure there's medical jargon to soften up how it sounds, but that was the simplified version, and I'm not a medical expert.

So, to make sure this was the case, I had to get violated three more times on top of my previous violation that day. They had to insert a tube into my butt to pump air into the pouch, to make sure that again no leaks or holes were there. I shudder to think what would have happened if there was a leak—would my pouch pop like a balloon? Probably not, because why else would they do this if that was the end result; still it was a terrifying thought. Perhaps that was the hypochondriac in me talking.

Tube number two was inserted a plasma-like gel that filled the pouch, and this had two purposes. Again, to make sure the pouch could hold waste without giving in or having leaks. Also, this plasma like gel lit up my pouch so I could get a CT scan done on me again to see what was going on inside. My fear of being put through the CT scan a second time was happening, on top of being violated on multiple instances.

The news came back great that day. No leaks in the pouch; it healed perfectly just like Dr. Gorfine had promised. The CT scan showed no bleeding. Everything was healed and looking good. There wasn't a shred of bad news administered on this day, and yet I felt totally deflated. I felt like a patient again, and that didn't sit well with me. Having doctors shove tubes and scopes up my butt, putting me through CT scans, and being probed made me feel sub-human even though I wasn't being treated that way. My doctors were compassionate—hell, they were even happy for me that day. They knew it was good news, but mentally, I was exhausted.

As we left the doctor's office, my mom and my dad began to spread the good news. They called my grandparents and told them that instead of mid-October, I was going to be operated on in two weeks on September 28. My whole family rejoiced as my phone was blowing up with text messages and phone calls from loved ones celebrating the good news. Except, I still wasn't that thrilled; I mostly sat quiet as they paraded on. Once we got home from the city that day, I went straight to bed. I knocked out after what was probably one of the more mentally draining days, I had throughout the entirety of my health battle.

## THE LAST ONE

As the weeks went by, I prepared for the second surgery. The preparation this time around was different in some ways and similar in other ways. I didn't have to sterilize my abdomen like I did for my first surgery. I had to stop eating a day before the surgery to make sure I was empty, so I was still empty but at least this time I didn't have to drink a laxative that smelt like gasoline. Which made sense because if I drank a laxative in my current condition, I'd probably wind up in the hospital for a whole different reason.

One of the things that remained the same were the nerves I felt the night before and on the morning of the surgery. I went to bed with a similar angsty feeling deep in my gut just like the first time. Text messages lit up my phone, this time with a more encouraging tone.

*Tomorrow is the big day! One more surgery and it's on the road to normalcy.*

*No more bag after tomorrow! How exciting, saying a prayer for you.*

*Good luck tomorrow, Michael. This is the easier one.*

I sat in my bed reading the texts, and although this time I had something to be excited about, it was still unnerving to have to be put under not knowing what would transpire. I was told by Dr. Gorfine this surgery would be significantly shorter than the first one. The first surgery was an extensive nine-hour operation; this one wouldn't take longer than the movie *Rush Hour*.

We had to wake up at the crack of dawn just like the first operation. My family always scheduled that appointment time for surgery because my mom believed they would be well rested and on their A-game. If it were me doing the surgery at 7 a.m., I would be snoozing on the job, but I guess that's why they get paid the big bucks and I don't.

We arrived at Mount Sinai once again to endure the same check in process. Sit in a waiting room here, recite my proce-dure and surgeon back to the hospital staff, get a fancy wrist band slapped on me, and move along to the next room. This time when I was in the pre-op room, I didn't need any drugs to ease my nerves. I was just ready to get the damned ostomy bag off me. While sitting in my bed waiting, I suddenly real-ized I was embodying the characteristics of that woman I saw the first time around who was unflinchingly reading her book as if she was just waiting to get her nails done or something. I wasn't reading a book, but I also wasn't lost in my thoughts scrambling to try and stop myself from shaking with fear. This time it was a more *fuck it let's get this over with* attitude. Maybe that woman on that day was in a similar spot; maybe she was having her fuck-it moment as well.

Dr. Gorfine came in dressed in all black scrubs this time around. My dad and I joked that he had his "Dark Knight" scrubs on since we are huge fans of the Christopher Nolan *Batman* trilogy—plus, it gave me a much-needed chuckle.

"Alright, Michael, this is it, the grand finale," Dr. Gorfine joked with his voice muffled through his pink surgical mask.

I sat propped up in the bed, looking more energetic and attentive then the first time around. "Let's get this sucker off of me."

Dr. Gorfine nodded. "This one should be an easier one. When you wake up, the pain should be nothing like the first time."

"I sure hope so, Doc," I said, half joking and half serious.

After we had our brief discussion, it was time to whisk me away. Gorfine was working without his assistant on this one, so he didn't need to wait for anyone. He was the commander and chief of this operation. He pushed me down the hallway, offering some more of his dry humor to lighten the mood, although this time I didn't really need it as much.

When we got into the operating room, it was the same sight as last time. Shiny silver equipment everywhere, reflections beaming around every corner. Medical assistants methodically strapping me onto the freezing cold operating room table that made the hairs throughout my body stand at attention once again. Then the mask was put over my face and the burning first breath of the anesthesia made me drowsy. By the second breath, I was out.

# CHAPTER 15

# AFTERMATH OF SURGERY NO. 2

---

When I woke up this time around, it was nothing like the first time. I didn't feel like I was in a dream; I was fully aware of my surroundings. I woke up in the operating room, still on the bed that I was initially strapped into. I felt refreshed almost, like I had taken a satisfying nap. The surgical team was taking the straps and tubes off of me, and some of them were surprised to see me awake. In the corner of the room, I saw Dr. Gorfine sitting on an office chair with his legs crossed and head down answering a text message or something on his phone.

He looked up from his lap to see I was awake. "Somebody's up early. How are you feeling?"

*Good question—how was I feeling?* I thought about it for a second. I wasn't in splitting pain anywhere in my body. I didn't feel sick in my stomach or abdomen area. To be completely honest, I didn't feel like I got operated on.

"Good Doc, I'm not in…," I was hesitant to say the rest hoping I wouldn't jinx myself, "…any pain."

I began to fumble around my abdomen area to lift up my gown and see the site of the surgery. Where the stoma used to be was a thick white gauze pad. No tubes hanging out the side of my abdomen, no tubes in my butt, and I didn't have an IV or a catheter. Things were going significantly better than the first time around, and I was a happy camper.

That was until I began to prop myself up more, and that was when I felt the first wave of pain. It wasn't life changing pain, but it was enough to make me go "ouch" and let out a wince.

"Yeah, don't get too carried away there. I still did some work on you. You'll feel pain, but it should be much more manageable then the first time," Dr. Gorfine said in a slow-your-roll tone.

I nodded, realizing I should've known better. "Well, it definitely is much better than the first time."

After our brief dialogue, the surgical team lifted me up from the operating room table to a stretcher and sent me to the post-op room. Once I was set up, my family was permitted into the room.

My mom and dad walked in, saw me in the bed, and let out a warm welcome. "Hey bud, how are you feeling?"

I was a bit more tired at this point, but I still felt good. "Much better than the first time. It doesn't hurt that much."

My mom made a shocked face that quickly morphed into a grin. "That's great news! What does it feel like?"

"Well, it kind of feels like a sports injury," I lifted my hand up and began pointing to the gauze area. "Only that area hurts when I move it. Everything else feels fine."

"That's good. Did you see Dr Gorfine yet?" my dad asked.

"Yeah, I saw him in the operating room after I woke up."

My dad looked shocked. "You woke up in the OR?"

"Yeah, Dr. Gorfine had a similar reaction. I guess that's a good thing."

My mom and dad looked at each other, shrugged, and said, "Guess so. We're off to a good start it seems."

After we chatted for a little, the effects of the anesthesia and the operation caught up with me and I took a little cat nap. I'm not sure how long I was out for, but it couldn't have been for too long. Though the surgery didn't completely wipe me out, it wasn't like I was going to tap dance out of the hospital on my own will with all the energy in the world.

When I awoke, my vision was blurry and distorted, and I saw a black blob in my frame. I blinked a couple of times, wiped some crud from my eyes, and realized the black blob was Dr. Gorfine in his "Dark Knight" scrubs.

"Ah, perfect, he's waking up again, Doc," my dad said, grabbing Dr. Gorfine's attention.

"Getting some beauty rest, eh?" he said jokingly.

I smiled. "Yeah, it's not easy maintaining these looks."

"Well, while things are looking good, and they are looking good," Dr. Gorfine said directly to my mom and dad, "I have to remind you guys we are still far from over. Things can still go wrong. I don't believe they will, but still."

"We understand. Thank you again Dr. Gorfine for everything you've done," my mom said.

"Don't thank me yet," he said modestly. "Your room is almost ready so you guys should be up soon. Be patient, you're going to have your own room this time."

Though rooming with Dimitri was a blessing in disguise, hearing I would have my own room was a relief. I knew this surgery would involve a lot more running to and from the bathroom, and for that, having my own room was nice. Not to mention that this time around we learned from our mistakes the first time, and we were getting me situated in the gastro unit. I was going to be in Dr. Gorfine's "stomping grounds," as he jokingly called them.

After an hour or so passed it was time for me to get wheeled up to my room. My family and I jokingly called it the "VIP room" because that is what it resembled. My room was located at the end of the hallway, and on the front of the door was "PATIENT: MICHAEL CAPRIO, SURGEON: DR. GORFINE." My bed was located on the left side of the room, and on the right side was an unoccupied bed, which my family used to rest on when visiting me. A nice thirty-some-odd-inch HDTV hung from the wall, which I watched college football on since it was the weekend. The view from my room, and the gastro unit in general, was a gorgeous overlook of Central Park.

I could tell after my introduction to the gastro unit that this was the right choice, and it should have been the call for the first time around. My condition and my operation are rare, and I was treated with more delicate care in gastro. The staff on the gastro floor specialized in patients with conditions similar to mine, so if I were to have an issue the nurses were only a couple steps away from giving me the care I need. Not to mention that since I was under Dr. Gorfine's care, I got a special type of treatment—at least it felt that way. Whenever nurses would enter the room, they would say how great of care I was under with Dr. Gorfine.

A major difference between the first surgery and the second was I had more freedom and independence this time around. I only had my IV pole and that was it. Not having multiple tubes going in and out of my body was liberating. My incision site was pretty gross, but not nearly as grotesque as the first time around. It was an oval shaped incision about the size of my thumb in length. It was about three inches wide, and it began to divide in the center. I had the gauze covering it, but you could see a shadow cast on the edges and the gauze in the middle wasn't sticking to anything. That's because the center of the wound was open and deep, almost like a valley with my skin on the edges of the gauze acting as the mountains. In the center of that valley, my wound was packed tight with more gauze, but between the cracks of gauze you could see the pulsation of my intestines. My wound was completely open, and for stomas, the wound had to close on its own without stitches or sutures. So, needless to say, it was quite the sight to see.

Dr. Gorfine was being cautious because, although this surgery wasn't as graphic as the first one, it was extremely meticulous. This surgery Dr. Gorfine described as putting the pipes, or plumbing, back together. When he described what he did, he said he had to connect the ends of my intestines back together. He said it was like putting two pieces of wet tissue paper back together. That wound had to heal, and the intestines had to heal perfectly, which would explain why he was so cautious and why I was watched so carefully. It also explained why my wound was packed so tightly with gauze to prevent infections. This surgery was more or less a waiting game to see what would happen when my intestines "woke up."

This was another thing Gorfine and his surgical team explained to me during my second time in the hospital. As a defense mechanism, they told me my intestines shut down when they are touched. No more waste is going through them, all operations are halted, and they are essentially asleep. At least that's how it was described to me. Upon doing my own research to confirm this phenomenon, it's called post-operative ileus or bowel paralysis.[28] The scientific reasoning for why this happens is because monocytes attribute to the inflammation of the intestines at first, but then begin to clean up the damaged tissue, which results in the inflammation decreasing.[29] So, I was essentially waiting for the monocytes to do their job. Scientists have been trying to figure out ways to speed up this transition from cleaning to normalcy, so I guess walking was something they figured might help.

The gastro ward had a room and a walkway on the opposite end of my room. The walkway had windows on both sides, and you had a perfect view of Central Park. The view was quite the incentive to take the needed walk, plus there wasn't much to do, and I felt good enough to do it. When I had enough energy, my mom and I would walk to the end of the walkway and observe the people as they enjoyed a beautiful fall day in the park. If I was a bit winded and still wanted to take in the view, we would plop down in the "view room" as we called it.

Though I felt as if I could eat normal food, I was still being monitored cautiously. I had a bland diet of water, ice chips, and the IV stand to start on the first twenty-four hours. For patients like me, everyone's intestines wake up and react differently. Much like the first time, they were expecting me to throw up when my intestines finally decided to contribute to the cause again.

The first day, I was monitored closely, and my family and I were waiting for the bomb to drop. Except it never did. Day

---

28   Ku Leuven, "Mechanism behind Bowel Paralysis after Surgery Revealed," ScienceDaily, June 20, 2017.

29   Ibid.

one was a pretty normal day. I spent it walking around limitedly, watching college football with my family. I would've liked to try some real food, but I understood from my first go that everything is done for a reason. If they wanted me to take it slow, then we were going to do that.

## DAY 2

The second day I was greeted in the morning by Dr. Gorfine and his surgical team, which was a ritual to start and end each day. His team was comprised of two women and two men who resembled a medical version of the Avengers.

"How are we feeling this morning, Michael?" Dr. Gorfine asked, smiling. "Did a lot of walking yesterday—you seem to not be in much pain."

"Yeah, the pain isn't bad at all—like a sports injury is how I described it to my mom."

My mom looked up at Dr. Gorfine. "Yeah, he's doing well, better than we expected."

My mother's face went from happiness to concern as she loaded up her next question, "But he hasn't gone to the bathroom yet. When should that start exactly?"

"Good question. That's pretty much what we're monitoring. We are going to upgrade you from the water diet to some Jell-O—nothing crazy, but something a bit more of substance."

"When do you think I can have real food?" I asked, salivating for a real meal.

"Probably your last day here, maybe tomorrow. We'll have to see how things go. Remember to keep on walking."

As they were wrapping things up, a member from his surgical team began to change my gauze. Once the gauze was replaced, they went on their merry way, and it was another day of waiting for me. During the morning I felt fine and continued to walk in between my Jell-O and water breaks. After lunch time though, I began to feel a bit sick. As I was laying down in bed watching the college football games, I felt a bit chilly.

I snuggled the blankets up over my arms and torso. "Hey Mom, can you turn the heat up in here?"

My mom shot a concerned look back at me. "Sure, are you feeling ok?"

I thought about how I felt for a second, then responded, "Well, I don't have aches or anything. My stomach doesn't hurt. I'm cold right now."

My mother got up and pushed the heat up. "Okay, but if you feel worse let me know so we can get a nurse in here."

First it was the chills, but after an hour or so, the aches decided to tag in and join forces. I laid under the covers, shivering. "Mom," my teeth chattering in between breaths, "I think we should call a nurse now."

My mom quickly shuffled to the nurse button and pressed it. "Relax, they'll figure this out. This is probably expected," she said reassuring me.

The nurse came in and attended to my fever. She pulled out the thermometer, stuck it in my mouth, and took it out after the beeps came in. She looked at it through her black-rimmed glasses. "He has a fever, but this is pretty common with procedures like his. It's to be expected. I got something for him to help in the meantime."

She left the room and returned back with a needle, which was promptly injected into my shoulder.

"If it gets any worse, give us a buzz. Right now, it isn't too high. If he starts running a high fever let us know ASAP," she said before she left.

This part of the recovery process in the hospital was a bit nerve-wracking. *Was this expected or was it going to get worse because of something happening beneath the surface?* I guess I had to wait and see, besides I had faith in Dr. Gorfine. I tried reminding myself that this happened the first time, and I have been under close watch for this precise reason.

After the shot was administered, the fever and aches got a bit better. It was still there, but not as dire and uncomfortable as before. As the evening rapidly approached and we entered dinner time, the fever symptoms were accompanied with nausea. My stomach began to rumble and twist and turn. I knew this feeling all too well.

"Mom, I don't feel so good," I said belching afterwards.

My mom's protective instincts kicked in as she looked nervous but attentive. "What is it? What's wrong?"

"Get a nurse to get a bucket or something." I burped into my fist and held my stomach in agony. "It's like the first time." I couldn't finish the sentence before another burp came up.

My mom knew what I was talking about and ran into the hall to get a nurse's attention. She came back with the same nurse from before, who gave me a white bucket I could throw up into. I grabbed the bucket and began to dry heave. Nothing was coming up but at this point I wanted it to come up so it could be over with. My mom sat beside me, rubbing my back and looking up at the nurse.

"Is he going to be okay? Is this normal?"

"This probably means his intestines are starting to become responsive again. Nothing out of the ordinary, unless it persists for a day or so."

The waiting game started again—this time we were monitoring how much I was going to be throwing up. I spent the rest of the second night huddled over a bucket, dry heaving and vomiting that vile green bile again as my mom consoled me, rubbing my back. It brought back memories to our original experience in the hospital. The sounds of me dry heaving were pretty loud, and I can imagine, from my mom's perspective, pretty worrisome. But it wasn't as bad as round one. This episode was different because it persisted all night, with nothing coming up the majority of the time. The last time around it all came up, and it was immediate relief afterwards. In the end, I think I still would have rather puked it all up in one fair shot like the first time. Because of this, I got little to no sleep and was pretty drained going into the next day.

## DAY 3

On the morning of day three, I was greeted at the crack of dawn by the medical Avengers team led by Dr. Gorfine himself. This morning, he wasn't joking with me initially. I think he heard through the grapevine I had a rough night.

"We feeling a bit better this morning?" he asked with a serious tone.

I rubbed my eyes and let out a yawn. "Tired, better than last night though."

"A lot of vomiting last night?"

"Not as much vomiting as it was dry heaving," my mom said, interjecting herself into the conversation.

Dr. Gorfine didn't look rattled or frustrated. "Obviously, today we are going to monitor you to make sure that doesn't happen again." His expression changed to happy. "But I think all that walking finally woke everything up. Today you'll have your first real meal to see how that goes."

My eyes lit up. "Like no Jell-O, no ice chips, actual food?"

He laughed. "Yes, actual food, and if that goes well then you'll be out of here tomorrow."

My mom and I looked at each other shocked. "Tomorrow?" we both said in unison.

"Yes, if things go well with the food you'll be out of here tomorrow. Isn't that exciting?"

I snapped out of my shocked expression. "Yeah, that's great. I wasn't expecting it so soon."

What I had originally thought would be a week or so in the hospital only turned out to be a three-day weekend. I didn't see this coming, so with my newfound excitement, my mom and I took a trip over to the view room. We spent a lot of the day continuing to walk and stay hydrated. Then, by dinner time, it was time to try my first sliver of actual food.

I still had an ultra-bland diet compared to what I eat nowadays. But, for the moment, this might as well have been a five-star dinner. It consisted of apple sauce, turkey, and a baked potato. From Jell-O and ice chips to turkey and apple sauce, I was living large. I was still a bit scared to eat because I didn't know how my body was going to react to it, though my mind was begging to devour it without much thought. I salivated as I punctured the turkey with my fork and lifted it up to my mouth. The food hit my tongue, and my tastebuds exploded with thanks while they savored the luxury of actual food for the first time in days.

I took my time with eating, and the nurses at the hospital were flooding me with all sorts of new information. I got a visit from someone who worked under Gorfine. She was a middle-aged nurse with brown curly hair, glasses, and sun-kissed skin. She came in, introduced herself, and was holding a clipboard in her right hand. "I know it's tempting to shove the food down as fast as possible, but you want to take this *slow,*" she said, spelling it out for me.

I chewed the food methodically and looked on for more information.

"Chewing slow is important to make sure it's as broken down as possible. Also, chew with your mouth closed for now so that there isn't as much gas. You want to take it easy this time around; your intestines have been through a lot."

I swallowed cautiously as she made me a bit nervous. "Is there anything else I should know?"

She put the clipboard back at her side. "Yes, yes there is. Take it slow with your diet, don't willy-nilly; eat anything you want. Also, it might be in your best interest to avoid any spicy foods. First month is going to burn enough as is."

*Burn enough as is—what the hell?*

"Uhm…what exactly does that mean?"

"Your large intestine takes the enzymes and acids out of your waste, your small intestine removes some but not all. So, until your body gets used to it, your bottom might be considerably sore," she said honestly with a pained expression on her face.

I sat there, not really sure how to digest what she had told me. I couldn't find what to say.

"It'll be okay. It's going to hurt for the first month or so. It's a process, as I'm sure you know."

*Oh, I know alright. Wish it could be over already.*

After she left, I finished my dinner slowly and waited for the worst to happen. Except nothing happened…I was repeatedly being warned by my doctors and nurses that at some point I was going to erupt like Mt. St. Helens. They were waiting for me to go to the bathroom, but I didn't have to. Part of me was concerned; I felt fine. No stomach gurgling, no urge to go, I was walking around after to try and make it happen. I forced myself to go thinking something was wrong, and nothing. My mom and I were a bit concerned but figured maybe we would get a break this time. Maybe this time around was going to be a super easy and fast recovery to out all the suffering I already endured.

Later that night, I was visited by two nurses and a doctor from Gorfine's surgical team. They debriefed me that I would be leaving tomorrow morning or early afternoon if I was still feeling well, which was a shock considering we were only in the hospital for three days. They removed the gauze that was packed together inside my wound, which was quite uncomfortable because they had to reach inside and pull it out. It didn't hurt as much as I thought it would because there aren't many nerve endings inside where the wound was. At least that's how it was explained to me.

After they took the gauze out, the inside of the wound was now completely visible. Inside the indent in my abdomen you could see the slimy red lining of my tissue, and if you looked close enough, you could see the pulsating of my intestines, which was grotesque at first but then became oddly fascinating to look at. My dad thought it looked really cool; my mom, not so much. Myself, I was somewhere in the middle. After that, it was time to hit the hay that night.

## DAY 4

I was still feeling good, no bathroom urges or issues. When I woke up, I was greeted by a jovial Dr. Gorfine, by himself this time.

"Hey Michael, you ready to say goodbye to this place for good?" he asked, smiling. Then, he began to read my shirt. I had on my "Hopatcong Class of 2015" shirt. He looked intensely at it as he tried to pronounce the name. "Ho…puh… cong?" He looked at me for approval of the pronunciation.

I laughed. "Ho…PAT…cong. You were close though. Nobody ever gets it right."

He shrugged. "I tried. Any questions you got for me? Feel good?"

"Yes, I do feel good but that's also drawing some concern for me and Mom. We were told I'd be going to the bathroom a lot, and I haven't gone yet. What's going to happen?"

"Well, you will be going a lot, I can promise you that. It is a part of the process, and it's taking just a little longer for you. This happens with some patients, but it's totally normal. I wouldn't expect it to be like this forever. There's a chance, but very marginal."

*Should've figured that was too good to be true.*

I sat in the bed digesting what he said. "So, what should I do, you know, to ensure I recover to the best of my ability?"

"Like the nurses said, be easy with the diet at first. Don't eat fast; chew thoroughly. When the time comes where you'll be going to the bathroom a lot, my best advice to you is to hold out as long as you can. If at first, it's only for a couple of seconds," he used his hands to demonstrate this next part, "this will stretch the pouch. The longer you hold, the bigger it gets, and the less you'll have to go to the bathroom in the long run. That is the best advice I can give you for this one."

I nodded my head. I was going to follow his instructions to a T. I kept repeating to myself in my head to keep holding when the time came.

"So, we're out of here today?" I asked with a smile on my face.

"I'd say so. You can walk and eat, no problem. We need this bed for folks who actually need it," he said jokingly.

"Well, I sure don't need it. Home sounds nice."

"I'd start getting your stuff situated. I'll start the process of getting you out of here."

He left the room, and it was time to leave the hospital once and for all. My mom began to pack our stuff up. My aunt had made shirts with the words "SHIT HAPPENS" on them. It was a plain black T-shirt with those words in all caps and bold white lettering. I changed into that shirt for when I was getting ready to leave the hospital. The nurses and doctors got a kick out of it and thought it was funny.

After I changed, I went into the bathroom to shave. I had been trying to grow out my facial hair during this time. I hadn't shaved since my first surgery on July 10. My beard was patchy on the sides but grew in fine under my lip and on my chin. My mom wanted me to shave it all off since we wouldn't be having any more operations. As I sat in the bathroom looking in the mirror, I had a change of heart. I was going to shave, but I didn't want to get rid of it all. I wanted to try something new, something new for a new chapter in my life. So, I shaved the sides and kept a goatee. It was actually thicker than I anticipated it to be. After I was done wiping the shaving cream on my face, I looked in the mirror and smiled back at my new image.

I walked out of the bathroom and turned the corner.

"So, what do ya think?" I asked with my arms stretched apart posing like a goof.

My mom looked at me for a second to see what the hype was about, and then she smiled. "I actually like it. It's different."

"Figured I'd try something new since we're leaving this place behind."

"Not a bad way to look at it. Now let's get out of here."

Everything was packed up, and when it was time, I was dismissed by Gorfine's surgical team. I was able to walk out of the hospital this time on my own power. The car ride home was still bumpy and uncomfortable but not nearly as troublesome as the first time. I was doing so well my parents stopped at GameStop to treat me to a video game of my choosing. I was able to walk in and pick it out no problem. When we got home that day, I spent the rest of the night playing *NBA 2K*, not feeling sick at all.

I started thinking to myself, if this is all that's going to happen then this is going to be a cakewalk. The first day home concluded, and it was another smooth day. What I didn't know is I was on a delay, and the eating was about to catch up to me. I just didn't know it yet.

## CHAPTER 16

# ROUND 2, FIGHT!

———

I woke up the following morning feeling as good as the night before. My surgery site was still tender and sore, but manageable. I didn't have the bathroom issues everyone was preparing me for—not yet. My mom made me breakfast, which was two pancakes, four eggs sunny side up, and a glass of strawberry banana juice. I ate it with no problems again, which was beginning to shock my mom and my grandma.

"He hasn't started going yet?" I heard my grandma ask as my mom had her on speaker phone. I was in the living room watching TV, and two rooms to the left, my mom was sitting at the dining room table talking with my grandma.

My mom responded in a hushed tone, "No, he's only gone twice but that's because he feels he should be going by now. Do you think…." My mom paused. "Do you think this is going to be it?"

"Oh, I'm not sure about that, but who knows, a lot has happened in medicine since we were operated on," my grandma said, her voice echoing from the dining room. I began to walk into the kitchen, the neighboring room, and cupped my ears to get a better listen.

"I know but still, nothing at all? That's got me a bit more concerned."

I pieced together what they were talking about and came around the corner into the dining room.

"I feel fine, ya know," I said implying I heard the entirety of their "private" conversation.

"Hi Michael, how are you doing sweetie? We're concerned is all," my mom said, startled at my sudden presence.

"I know you guys are, but maybe this time will be easier for me. I don't get the need to panic. This is good news, right?"

My mom looked back at me and responded before my grandma could. "It's not that we aren't happy, but you had a lot of work done. We all had to go through this next phase."

I shrugged, "Well, maybe I got lucky for once."

*Jinx, it suddenly hit me at once.* My stomach began to gurgle and get tense. I put my hand over my gut and hunched over as my abdomen contracted in a spasm-like manner. My mom looked worried and grabbed my hand. She grabbed the phone. "Mom, I think it's starting to happen."

My grandma collected herself. "Okay Mar, don't panic. Remember, we were waiting for this to happen."

I remembered Dr. Gorfine's advice, saying it over and over in my head. *Hold as long as you possibly can—that's the best advice I can give you on this one.*

So I did, although the first time I could barely hold for ten seconds before I scurried off to the bathroom as my abdomen contracted with wave after wave of throbbing agony. I dashed away from the dining room table and ran to the bathroom abruptly leaving the conversation I wandered into. It felt as if the volcano had awoken from slumber, even though when I went to the bathroom, I barely got any relief. Next to nothing came out, and I know this isn't the most pleasant subject matter, but this was the reality I was now in. I couldn't figure out for the life of me how I was in such gastric distress and little to nothing came out. *What was causing that pain?* After I went to the bathroom the first time, the flood gates had opened, and I was now on a cycle of going to the bathroom every half hour for the rest of the day.

That's not an exaggeration either; the waves of spasms wouldn't go away anytime soon, and they were followed by bathroom visits that gave me no relief whatsoever. The first day of going to the bathroom was my body's way of catching up for the past three months of not going the usual route. After hours of running back and forth to the bathroom and not eating anything for the rest of the day because I was now officially petrified to eat, we needed an answer to put an end to this misery. We called Dr. Gorfine hoping maybe he could give us some answers to what was happening.

The way he explained it over the phone to me and my mom was that my body was essentially being potty-trained all over again. For eighteen years of my life, I went to the bathroom via the large intestine like everyone else. My body and organ systems were used to this way. But things were significantly different now, considering a major organ was now missing from my body. My body was confused and didn't know how to react to the new "plumbing" as Dr. Gorfine called it. He said it would take time for my body to become accustomed to this new plumbing system constructed inside of me, hence the incredibly painful spasms, and why little to nothing was coming out when I would go to the bathroom.

That pain I felt, those spasms, the contractions, all of it was because the pouch was expanding. It hadn't had any waste in it, and it was now being put to the test for the first time ever. If I wanted to eat the way I'm accustomed to eating, which is a lot, then I was going to have to endure this pain and stretch the pouch out. He further reinforced for me to hold as long as I can, even if for only a couple of seconds.

He ended the call telling us I should be taking Imodium before and after every meal so I can slow the bathroom trips down. I had to eat and take the Imodium, and I had to hold it in as long as possible. The first day I went twenty plus times, and I remember Dr. Gorfine saying on the phone twenty times is way too much. The medicine helped, but it's not like I noticed the impact of it initially. It took me from twenty times the first day to ten to fifteen times a day. For the first month, I had to keep tabs on what I ate daily so if something disagreed with me, we could find the culprit and discard it immediately. As strange as it sounds, we also had to keep tabs on how much I was going to the bathroom. This was to make sure I was improving and to make sure the number was decreasing daily.

When you go from twenty times in day one, to say fifteen in day two, you notice no difference if you aren't keeping tabs on the number of times you go in a day. It feels the same, still running back and forth to the bathroom, painful spasms, fear of eating food for the sake of spending the rest of the night in the bathroom. Needless to say, I was lucky to sleep for a handful of hours each night because I would be up every hour to be back in the bathroom. I was also lucky if I didn't have an accident, and accidents were unfortunately a regular thing for the first month. I wasn't exaggerating when I said I was being potty-trained all over again at eighteen years old.

I began to have my doubts during my second recovery, like the first one, but I internalized them this time instead of projecting them onto my friends and family. I wondered to myself during that first miserable week of being chained to my bathroom, *How will I ever be able to go out if this is what life is going to be like? How can I live a full life if I'm tied to a bathroom?* I countered these negative thoughts by trying to be tough and remembered Dr. Gorfine's advice, *Hold as long as possible.* Not only that, but I tried to remember the end result Dr. Gorfine promised me: his patients go two to six times a day.

I remember what my reaction in that first visit with him was, *How the hell am I going to adjust to two to six times a day in the bathroom?* That sounded like a fantasy in this moment, a fantasy I hope would come true. Everything Dr. Gorfine told me had come true, and the first surgery was the most difficult one, and he got me through. His work was so good I recovered in three months after a nine-hour operation that took away my large intestine and reconfigured my small intestines. If he could do that, then this would be fine.

Having said that, it wasn't easy for me mentally. My second surgery inflicted a whole bunch of mental blocks on me. For one, I was terrified of eating in the beginning. Eating meant my intestines would start digesting food and that would end in multiple bathroom trips, painful spasms, and a sore bottom. That wasn't worth it; I would rather not eat. But my mom was a meal dictator making sure I ate three squares a day, no matter how much pushback I gave her. Suddenly, eating real food, which was joyous in the hospital, was now a chore—much more of a chore than my first surgery. At least when I had the bag, my bottom was spared from the carnage. I was starting to see why certain patients like the bag as opposed to what I have.

Then, I began to think about all the activities I might want to do once (or if) I fully recovered. Activities like playing basketball at the park, going for hikes, and camping for starts. These activities began to weigh on my mind because there isn't a bathroom during events like this, at least not a bathroom I'd be comfortable using. This was another phobia I would have to overcome: using public restrooms.

I began to feel for the first time the limitations I might have on my life moving forward. As these thoughts manifested themselves, I got a bit discouraged. Yes, I didn't have the bag on me anymore, which was great, and I no longer had to worry about it. But now I had to worry about if my stomach would hold up when I went out. In a way, I guess the two situations are a bit more similar than I realized initially.

I began to lose trust in my body for the first time in my life, and this anxiety doubled with my OCD. It was now an obsession, the thought of going out and having a bad bathroom night. If it did happen, it probably wouldn't be the end of the world, but it was still embarrassing for me to think about the potential of it happening. *What happens if I'm playing pick-up basketball and those God-forsaken spasms start persisting*? I would have to leave in a hurry to find a bathroom, and certainly people would notice.

The first two days had passed, and they were brutal on my bottom. The third day was more or less the same result. It was at least October, so horror movies were on every other channel. The channels that didn't have horror movies on had post-season sports. So, I had entertainment in between my bathroom trips for what it was worth.

I sat on the couch, lying on my side as my bottom was burning up. I had on the MLB post-season games, trying to take my mind off as I watched the excitement of playoff baseball. The crowd was going wild; the Yankees weren't even in it this year. I was watching to distract myself from the bad thoughts that began festering inside me and how much pain I was in. My mom walked out of her room to check on me.

"Hey." She looked at me laying on the couch with her arms crossed. "I know you don't feel like things improved between yesterday and today, but they did."

I looked at her with a blank face. I wasn't buying it. "Sure doesn't feel like it."

My mom walked into the kitchen and grabbed the bathroom tally sheet. "Well." She began to smirk and point at the tallies. "According to our shit chart, you're down by five today. Doesn't seem like much, but it is an improvement. The Imodium is working."

I knew she was making a cute gesture to point fun at our ridiculous circumstances, so I smirked back. "Yeah, at this rate I'll be at the coveted two to six mark by the time the years over."

My mom knew I was joking but tried to wash away some of my pessimism. "You're down five times in one day, sweetie. It'll be better quicker than you expect. Remember the first time around?"

She was right, and I knew it. I was down a little bit in my head, wrestling with the uncertainties of the future, but that was normal. At least that's what I had told myself. I was grieving and undergoing a massive change in my life three short months after another massive change. So sure, doubts were going to happen. I was going to have down moments where I was scared and unsure; that's part of being human. I acknowledged my feelings this time around and was able to *live* with them. I wasn't ignoring them, pushing them to the side, or blaming myself for feeling this way anymore. I accepted my situation and my emotions as they were. No sugar coating, no dismissing, just acceptance—and that made all the difference this time around.

Without sounding too redundant, this was the daily struggle I lived with for basically the entire month of October. It was the same thing every day for the most part. I would struggle to get a couple hours of sleep running back and forth from the bathroom all night. Then after I accepted, I wasn't going to sleep much more, my mom would make me break-fast which I dreaded. I dreaded eating in general because eating meant that the bathroom cycle from hell was about to start. My mother would then force the three-square meals down my throat. I would spend my time when I wasn't in the bathroom on the couch watching horror movies holding off as long as I possibly could. Reflecting back on it, it probably wasn't the best idea to watch scary movies while I had loose bowels, but luckily, we had no accidents on the couch.

Some days were worse than others, it would fluctuate. The good news was, after the Imodium became a regular part of my daily routine before every meal, I never hit the twenty mark again. That was a one-day deal and a personal record yet to be broken, thank God. The first week was hell, and I remained in the double digits for the entirety of the week. It was exhausting; I couldn't wait to have a restful night sleep more than anything. Sure, the burning butt and intestinal spasms were as horrible as they sounded, but a week without proper rest can make you a bit delusional.

The difference between this week of hell, however, was I didn't give up hope. I saw from the first surgery how things went from totally hopeless, to suddenly having a glimmer of hope. I didn't get all of my hope back when it came time for my second surgery, but I got *some* of it back and that was huge. That was enough to give me reason to believe things would get better this time around. Not to mention, I wasn't naive, part of me was hoping for a miraculously easy recovery this time around but I wasn't banking on it. I knew once the running to the bathroom began that the first week would be the roughest. My mindset this time around was to wait it out and, most importantly, follow Dr. Gorfine's golden rule of hold as long as possible.

As I rinsed and repeated my daily routine for the first treacherous week, things began to get a little better moving forward. Not significantly enough to where I trusted going out in public with my friends. But I was able to enjoy meals without rushing to the bathroom in the middle or toward the end of them. I was also able to enjoy ten minutes to a half hour sometimes, if I was lucky, of down time in between meals before the bathroom trips started piling up. This small sliver of things getting better was equivalent to that small sliver of hope I had during the first surgery when I was able to drink coffee again for the first time, or when I was able to drive without a donut under my butt. These were small steps, but they were enough once again to give me reason to believe. Patience was ultimately the most important virtue I learned during both my trips in the hospital. It takes a while for things to start moving in the right direction. You have to be patient and pay attention to the small signs. The tiny pieces to the big puzzle finally started to come together.

# PART V

# THE OPEN ROAD

# CHAPTER 17

# THANKFUL

---

The weeks following got progressively better. My short breaks of relief I had after meals, along with the enjoyment of eating again, were now complimented with fewer bathroom trips. I began to learn the signs from my new plumbing and my body began to adapt. I was learning signs of indigestion, foods that worked, foods that didn't work, and time periods in the day where my stomach wouldn't be reliable. I began to pick up on these signals my body would give me through sensations within my digestive track. I quickly learned how to manage my body. *Isn't it amazing how miraculously the human body can adapt?*

I had to learn how to live with my new system, while managing my lifestyle and diet so I didn't get myself sick. Examples of bad choices that lead to me getting sick, which still hold true today, are eating a reckless amount of carbs and not getting a serviceable amount of steps in. If I lay in bed all day, and ate carbs, that's a recipe for disaster. If I lived on carbs for a week and didn't do much running or walking, I could potentially give myself a blockage. Staying active and incorporating a well-balanced diet is my best bet at keeping myself in optimal shape. If I let my diet slip, then I could get backed up for weeks. Yes, *weeks,* which is something I didn't think was possible until recently.

At the time of this writing, we are living through the coronavirus pandemic. Needless to say, we haven't done much stepping during this time, especially in the beginning. Combine that with the stress eating of carbs and I backed myself up for two weeks of feeling bloated, constipated, and sick. So, five years later when the majority of my days are good, I still learn to not lose track of staying active and eating healthy.

This isn't a discouraging sign to me at all; I'm used to being on top of my health and keeping my body happy. It takes work and sometimes that slips away from me. We're all human, and in these beginning parts of figuring my body out I experienced more highs and lows with keeping myself managed. As time would go on, I became much better at managing my body.

Toward the end of October, I was able to have my first night out with my friends on Halloween. It wasn't anything crazy or out of the ordinary, but it felt nice to be able to go out again. My friends were talking about Halloween plans a week prior in our group chats. They were asking me if I felt good enough to hang out again, and my mom insisted I should get out if I can. It would do wonders for me mentally. It's not often my mother would convince me to go to a house party and not vice versa. So, I decided to have a fuck-it moment. A couple days before Halloween my friends wanted to go to the Halloween store to get costumes. The costume of choice was two priests and a friar. We decided to be the holy trinity this specific year.

When Halloween night came around, I was a bit nervous getting ready at my house. I had better control over my body then at the beginning of the month, there was no doubt. But I hadn't attended a social event yet quite like this. There was a lot of firsts that were going to happen tonight. It was going to be the first time in a long while a lot of people had seen me. A lot had changed, and I was still concerned with my diminished appearance. I wasn't as thin as the first time around, but my face was still thin as my cheeks looked sucked in. My eyes looked baggy and grey, and my skin was vitamin D deprived at this point in the fall. I was already looking particularly ghoulish to begin with—maybe I didn't need a costume after all. I was hoping no one would notice or point out my appearance, so that weighed a bit on my mind.

Another first was I hadn't left the sanctity of my home since the floodgates had opened in the beginning of October. I was going to be away from my glorious porcelain throne, my trusted bathroom that I had become chained to for the past month. I would get separation anxiety from a toilet, which sounds absurd, but it was oddly true. Have you ever tried to use a bathroom at a house party? *Disgusting.* It's a last option for any sane person. I've witnessed people use bushes in people's backyards as make-shift porcelain thrones. So, venturing out to do something where there was no bathroom made me a bit nervous.

It was the first night I was testing my body out, so to speak. It was a litmus test to see how the future would be. If I could get through the evening with no issues so soon after my surgery, then things will only get better from here on out. I was hopeful the situation would continue trending upward, but the potential for it going bad weighed on my mind.

I finished slipping into my priest robes for the night while I was in my room. I called my mom in for some assistance with the accessories to my costume. I also wanted her two cents. She walked in, and I put my arms out. "How do I look?"

My mom laughed at my costume. "You look ridiculous, but I'm sure that's what you're going for."

I rolled my eyes. "Well duh, the costume yes, but I meant me. How do I look?"

My mom adjusted the cross on my neck. "You look fine, sweetie. These are your friends. They want to see you and have fun. I doubt anyone is going to notice."

I sat there nodding, wanting to believe her but also still having my anxious doubts creep into my mind.

"Guess I won't know unless I find out." My dad came up from downstairs and saw me and my mom in the living room. He had caught a piece of our conversation.

"You're right, you won't find out until you go out. You need to have some fun, kid. Get out there." He came over and patted me on the shoulders a couple of times in true dad fashion.

My phone began to ring up with text messages as they were giving me words of encouragement to stop being on edge and to let my hair down and have some fun.

*You almost ready?*

*I'm ready to leave whenever Mike is.*

Well, the group chat was blowing up and they were ready for me to go pick them up. Needless to say, after everything I've been through, I wasn't drinking on this night. I wouldn't be drinking for a good little while after the surgeries. So, I was playing the role of driver; plus, I liked it. If something God forbid went wrong, I could leave when I needed too and not have to wait for a ride. That sentiment still holds true today.

Luckily for me the night was an encouraging sign of things to come. That worst-case scenario that was being painted in my head was simply not true. This was a start of me ignoring the outsider for good. His voice was still there but not nearly as loud and dominant as the past. His words held no power over me anymore as I didn't believe them. It was all lies. Perhaps they were true for a brief snapshot in time, but they certainly weren't the truth for the rest of my life.

I had people I haven't seen in months come up and talk to me. Some were happy to see me, and no one pointed out the diminished look in my appearance. People were more or less happy I was good and healthy—those who knew at least. A lot of people didn't know and, to my knowledge, they didn't know on this particular night. If they did it was never mentioned to my face, which I suppose is all that matters.

After Halloween went well, I was encouraged to inch out slowly into the real world. I began hanging out with my friends more frequently. I was doing stuff with my family with the trust of my body back. Going to my uncle's for the Giants football games, still paying visits to my grandma, and the occasional hangout at my friends' houses became part of my social life. It wasn't the normal social life from pre-surgery, but it was some semblance of a normal social life. Having those interactions—albeit they were different from the norm at first—was nice. It was again that sliver of hope, although this one was a bit bigger than the sliver, I was given a couple of weeks prior. This went from a sliver to a pretty healthy slice.

Being able to go out, from the comforts of home, was an always an adventure. Each time it went well, my confidence would grow. If I was out and about enjoying myself with no gastric issues, I would soak in all the beauties of the moment—simple beauties like being able to hold a long conversation over a slice of cake with a cup of coffee and not having to frantically run to the bathroom cutting the conversation short. That was a huge victory.

As I gained this newfound trust in my body, I was living again for the first time in a while. Life was different—I don't want to lose sight of that. But life had freedoms and individuality again. I still had my share of battles and hurdles to overcome, but I was able to become independent again. I was able to enjoy the holidays with my family again. Being able to eat a huge meal on Thanksgiving without being admitted to the hospital in gastric distress was lovely.

We were going to my aunt's lake house, which was luckily pretty close to us. It was about twenty-five minutes away, which is closer than going to other relatives' houses for the holidays. I had on my gray turtleneck sweater, with black joggers since they were comfy around my still tender belly, and formal gray shoes. I was actually dressed nice for the first time since my surgeries started. I was standing in front of the mirror in my closet, as I snapped my Apple Watch on and took in my appearance. It was nice to see myself getting closer to my original weight of 160 pounds. At this moment in time, I was probably floating around 150, and things were starting to shape together nicely. I wasn't super nervous about having a large dinner, cause at the least, I was with family. If something were to go wrong, I was with people who knew my situation.

After dinner was over that Thanksgiving, I sat on the couch in the living room watching football with the men of the family. The Cowboys were losing to the Panthers on this Thanksgiving, so for us Giant fans it was a happy occasion. My grandma came in the room with her bright red dress on.

"Hey Michael, you mind if I pry you away from the men for a second for a picture?"

Pop turned his head from the TV to Grandma. "You women and the pictures, can't you see this is football time?" my grandpa asked, joking with a smile.

My grandma put her hands on her hips and had a mischievous look on her face, "Well, for that answer you can be in the picture too, Don. Unless you don't want to take a pic with your grandchildren that is." She stuck her tongue out, flipping the blame on him.

Pop looked around at the other men in the room. "Let this be a lesson to the rest of you guys." The guys smiled back; their bickering was cute and amusing to the rest of us. Plus, my grandpa probably didn't want to admit it, but he did love taking family pictures. The women of my family do have a habit of picking inopportune times to take photos, however. Watching the Cowboys lose after digesting Thanksgiving dinner...not the best time.

Grandma had her photoshoot with all of us. A picture of me and her, then me, her, and Pop. Next up was me and my brother, then all of the grandchildren...you get the idea. Every combination you could think of was done, so that everyone got pictures, and no one got left out. After we were done with our photo session, I sat on the couch with my grandma and grandpa trying to look at the pictures we took.

I pointed at the phone screen. "Oh I like that picture of us, Gram. I don't look so thin."

She smiled back at me. "You look great, sweetie. You see how far you've come?"

I shrugged. "I guess you don't realize the progress you make along the way until you reflect on it."

Pop chimed in on the conversation. "Told ya, bud. Your grandmother, mother, and aunt all got through it. You were gonna be no different."

I reflected on the past couple months and remembered how distraught I was looking at my reflection in the bathroom after my first surgery. I remember being so embarrassed of my appearance throughout that first summer, and how a short month ago, on Halloween, I was still embarrassed. For the first time since this all started, I wasn't ashamed of how I looked. I wasn't 100 percent my old self yet, I still wanted to improve more, but it was a big moment in my progress. The fear of my surgery holding me back from gaining weight was also turning out to be a myth perpetrated by the outsider as I inched closer to my pre-surgery weight. *What else could I accomplish?*

I smiled. "I got a lot to be thankful for this year, don't I?"

My grandma put her hand on my back and rubbed it. "We all have a lot to be thankful for this year, Michael. A lot."

She was certainly right. There was a lot to be thankful for this year. I was thankful for my friends and acquaintances from my town who were understanding and nonjudgmental regarding my appearance, which I was insecure about at the moment. I was thankful for my incredible family for all the unconditional love and support they gave me, to build me back up when I needed it most. I was thankful for being able to see the first steps in my progress, with weight slowly being added back on and with gaining better control over my body.

# CHAPTER 18

# ACCOUNTABILITY

––––

## WORK AND JUDGMENT

I've seen both ends of the human condition. I saw the overwhelming compassion from my nurses, doctors, family, and friends. Then, as I began to assimilate back into the "normal" world, it meant that I was going to be thrown into the fire so to speak, the fire being society, and how cruel it can be sometimes. It started for me in small micro-doses when I got back to working again. I had just undergone life-changing surgery and getting back to the working world was an adjustment. I had to get used to being on my feet again, and that was one of the hardest things to adjust to. Standing hurt in the beginning, and my stamina was depleted. I used to be able to work a whole shift without taking a break, but that would be no more. My body simply couldn't handle that, and breaks would become necessary. Anyone who has ever worked a part-time job knows that taking breaks never sits well with the boss, no matter what the circumstances.

I had a particularly hard time once I started working at a liquor store after I left the coffee shop. One worker never got along great with me. He didn't get along with anyone at the job and was known for talking behind the employees' backs. This was brought to my attention before my first shift with him, and I was basically told to take whatever he says with a grain of salt. So, I did, and I thought our shift went smooth. He didn't complain about anything to my face, but I remembered my boss mentioning to me that he has a tendency to do this. So, it was no shock to me the next day when I came in and one of my co-workers proceeded to tell me about how he spent the entire night bitching about how I would always be in the bathroom. This particular co-worker knew my situation, so when he told me I just rolled my eyes. It wasn't public knowledge to everyone at the liquor store; I still liked some level of privacy. I didn't want to have to walk around and announce my business to the world if I didn't have too.

One afternoon, I was bringing up a box of beer from downstairs. Once I got to the top of the stairs, I plopped the box on the ground to wipe some sweat from my forehead. I was about to open the cooler door when I overheard my name in the background. I quietly tried to adjust my position so that I wasn't seen but could also hear what was being said.

"When I work with him, he's always in there. What could he possibly be doing in there?"

Without much context, I already knew what the conversation was about, and I rolled my eyes. Before I could get too frustrated my manager chimed in.

"He has a medical condition, you know."

Then an awkward silence filled the air, which I imagine he had a look of shame on his face.

"What is it?"

"It's not my business to tell you what *his* condition is. If you're so curious you can ask him yourself, but I don't think he's going to tell you."

*Thank you*, I exhaled followed by a grin. It was nice to hear someone stick up for me, and simultaneously it was nice to hear him get humbled. He never asked about my condition and never even brought it up to me again. As far as I know he didn't think I heard that conversation. I was happy for the gossiping to be silenced, and yes, my manager was correct; even if he asked me, he wasn't going to get debriefed.

The most notable time that I noticed this blatant lack of respect toward me was when I was serving at a local diner in a neighboring town. If you have ever worked as a server in any restaurant, you know the cutthroat and sometimes skeevy nature of the business. Double shifts, no breaks, late nights, rude customers, and then the server drama that was inevitable at any restaurant. When I worked at the diner, I was only working three nights a week because I was attending community college. I already had restaurant experience with my prior job at Buffalo Wild Wings. I wasn't working nearly that much in comparison to the other servers, some of which would be pulling forty-to-sixty-hour weeks. I was just there to work weekends, and the money I made from the three days I worked was plenty to get me by.

When I was feeling good, I was confident in my ability to work. Not to mention that I would take full advantage of it because I know it can evaporate. When I'm on my game, it is apparent to anyone who knows me. I will socialize and bounce all over the place, but when things start turning, that fades away. It's not easy to socialize and be happy when you're focusing all your energy fighting off gut-wrenching spasms in the abdominal area.

I would almost always start a shift out strong, with no worries. Then (and it varied each work shift) at some point, my stomach would start to turn. Usually, it would happen right around or after the dinner rush. Then I would panic. *Do I take a break and eat but potentially make my stomach worse? Or do I starve myself and not eat at all tonight?* It would always seem no matter what I chose, I would still find myself in pain and in the bathroom. I would try everything in my power to have a pain free shift with minimal bathroom trips. I would not eat before my shift, but that didn't work. I would eat a big early breakfast sometimes, and that didn't work either. The point being, I was trying to make it work—harder than most people who criticized me could even comprehend.

As time went on at the diner, rumors began to fly around. Restaurant gossip and drama is pretty standard for most places, but some places it can be a little much. The diner was a place where the drama was definitely over the top, and I have dealt with my fair share of work drama over the course of my life. A couple of servers were gossiping behind my back about my frequent bathroom trips. I never heard it directly, and honestly it blindsided me. Not to say that I was surprised necessarily that someone was gossiping, I was just surprised that I never caught wind of it. Nonetheless, after a long Saturday night we began wrapping up and collecting our money. It was almost one in the morning, which was the usual time we would be getting out. I sat at the counter as the owner sorted out all of our earnings for the night.

After he finished counting out the cash, he asked for me to stay behind, instructing the other servers to leave. I didn't know what was about to be dropped on me, but it was something obviously important. I never could have guessed the rumor flying around about me.

He brought to my attention that the other servers thought I was doing drugs or something suspicious in the bathroom throughout my shifts. *Can you believe that?* I was taken aback, and I just had to laugh it off. I've had people say petty things about my bathroom breaks, like at the liquor store, but none of that bothered me. It would deflect off of me; I always felt that it said more about them than me. But, to start a rumor about me doing drugs that got the owner's attention was just incredible to me.

Frustrated, I composed myself and gave the full disclosure to the owner, letting him know my medical history. He shook his head in disappointment at the rumor but was pleased to hear it was just that, *a rumor*. He explained to me that he had to confront me about it even though he didn't believe it because he's seen a lot in his years as a restaurant owner. If you hear rumors about an employee doing drugs in the bathroom, even if it seems far-fetched, you have to at least investigate the claim. He never accused me, and I wasn't mad at him, he was very understanding after hearing my situation. After that night, I told him that I was just waiting until the end of winter break to make my money for when I transferred schools, and I was out. In the meantime, he ignored the rumors after hearing my situation and defended me for my remaining time.

Perhaps the most frustrating aspect of this was no one realized how much I was holding back. Pretty much every shift I worked, at some point I was enduring a great deal of pain with a big ole customer service smile on my face. I had to suck it up and look like nothing was wrong or else it would affect my tips. If it didn't affect my tips then it would be noticed by my managers. I looked fine but underneath the surface, the reality was, I was hiding a great amount of discomfort that they had no idea about. I thought I did a good job keeping it mostly under control. Apparently, not as good as I realized since everyone had noticed something was up.

Shortly after this experience, I accepted the fact that not everyone was going to understand what I've gone through. I also accepted that people might be cruel toward me about it, as ridiculous as that sounded to me. It wouldn't be the last time that I have been unfairly judged because of it.

Friends and family often ask me how I deal with rumors and assumptions without getting angry or rattled, and the answer to me is simple. Any person who is quick to judge another person with an illness they can't control is battling some nasty demons of their own behind closed doors. Any person who can make fun of others so quickly without knowing the person, clearly is battling some insecurities of their own. Either that or they lack the wisdom and life experience to realize that all of us are battling some rather arduous things behind closed doors. Not everything is what it seems on the surface.

I never let it get the best of me though, even though taking the high road was difficult sometimes. I just had to try and remember everyone isn't perfect. I'm not perfect and have had my fair share of poor judgement moments in my life. I've let my emotions get the best of me before as you have read by now, so who am I to judge when I'm not perfect myself? Most of them didn't know, and I'm sure if it was ever brought to their attention, they'd feel some kind of remorse, even if it was just a tiny bit. At the end of the day, in high-stress jobs, sometimes people's emotions get the best of them. The point is, we're all not perfect, but it's something to be mindful of.

## EXERCISE

By 2016, I started watching YouTube videos on how to exercise for beginners and what to eat to gain mass. I was in research mode trying to gather routines for when I arrived at the gym and meals to plan for afterwards. Eventually, I stuck with it, applying some of that patience I learned about during my first surgery. I endured the pain associated with heavy lifting for the first time. You know, the struggle to take your shirt on and off the first couple days after a hard lift. I also endured the occasional embarrassment for being a beginner learning his way around the gym and learning correct form. But I'm glad I stuck with it because exercise was good for me in a lot of ways.

For starters, exercising did more mentally for me than it did physically. The physical stuff would come with time and consistent work, but the mental effects were immediate. Regular exercise eases depression and anxiety by releasing feel-good endorphins, natural cannabis-like brain chemicals (endogenous cannabinoids) and other natural brain chemicals that can enhance your sense of well-being.[30] It also requires your attention to be focused on the exercise at hand, preventing you from entering the negative cycle of feeding into your thoughts.[31] Not to mention the gym is a social environment with potential to meet other people, which is great for us being the social creatures we are. It also improves your confidence as time goes on and you begin to get in better shape. All of these things are *healthy* ways of coping with the stresses of life—not negative like doing drugs, drinking, or sulking in your own misery, much like I was doing. I had to go out of my comfort zone initially, especially with the nagging thought of, *Is my condition holding*

---

30  "Depression and Anxiety: Exercise Eases Symptoms," Mayo Clinic, Mayo Foundation for Medical Education and Research, September 27, 2017.

31  Ibid.

*me back?* The answer for those of you wondering was no, it hasn't held me back.

Other studies have shown that one hundred minutes a week of exercise combined with a healthy diet can decrease brain age by nearly ten years.[32] It improves cognitive flexibility and is an effective treatment for OCD, which I can confirm from my experiences that a good workout will take my mind down about ten notches when I'm wound up. [33,34] Perhaps one of the most interesting facts about regular exercise is how it stimulates "neurogenesis," which is the brains ability to generate new neurons.[35] If you stimulate these new neurons through mental or social interaction, following a workout, they can connect to other neurons and become integrated into brain circuits that help maintain their functions throughout your life.[36] This explains why people who hit the books after exercising, opposed to vegging out, are smarter.[37]

32  Victoria Allen, "Moderate Exercise Just Three Times a Week and Eating Healthy Can Take 10 Years Off Your Brain Age, Study Says," Daily Mail December 19, 2018.

33  Cell Press, "Physical Activity May Leave the Brain More Open to Change," ScienceDaily December 7, 2015.

34  Ana M. Abrantes et al., "A Pilot Randomized Controlled Trial of Aerobic Exercise as an Adjunct to OCD Treatment," General Hospital Psychiatry 49 November 2017: 51-55.

35  Daniel G. Amen MD, *The End of Mental Illness: How Neuroscience is Transforming Psychiatry and Helping Prevent or Reverse Mood and Anxiety Disorders, ADHD, Addictions, PTSD, Psychosis, Personality Disorders, and More* (Illinois: Tyndale Momentum,2020), 109.

36  Ibid.

37  Ibid.

All of this information is important for me, especially because the gut is known as the second brain. It is lined with 100 million neurons.[38] That's more neurons than the entirety of your spinal cord or peripheral nervous system.[39] I'd have to imagine that since I have no large intestine, I'm probably short fifty-some-odd million neurons in my gut. Being that I'm at a disadvantage in this category, exercise is even more imperative for myself. That's not even to mention all of the physical benefits it has done for me personally.

I was bad at drinking adequate amounts of water pre surgery. Now that I didn't have a large intestine, I dehydrated much quicker. If I didn't keep up with drinking water I could dehydrate and I was also at an increased risk of kidney stones, which are brutal. Any chance of absolving myself from that pain, I was going to take. Once I started exercising, water became my go-to drink. After a while, it became the only thing that quenched my thirst. I'm not sure if I started drinking water so much because my body simply needed it more, or if exercise played a role, but I think it was a bit of both.

Along with my intake in water, exercise helped my appetite. After I got into routinely working out, I was able to put down gargantuan portion sizes that I never thought I'd be able to eat before. My appetite is the best it's ever been in my life, and I could eat huge meals after my surgery once I discovered the beauty of exercising. As my grandpa put it, "I'm not sure what I'd rather do: feed him or clothe him."

---

38   Daniel G. Amen MD, *The End of Mental Illness: How Neuroscience is Transforming Psychiatry and Helping Prevent or Reverse Mood and Anxiety Disorders, ADHD, Addictions, PTSD, Psychosis, Personality Disorders, and More* (Illinois: Tyndale Momentum,2020), 135.

39   Ibid.

It also prevented me from getting constipated from inactivity. It became a necessary way to keep my mind and body in order. It was a way to have structure in my life, as well as a place to relieve my stress. All the other stuff I mentioned were bonuses I didn't think I was going to get. Above all, exercising was a good way to keep my body active and healthy after it had been through so much already. If there was a way to prevent future health issues after everything I endured, then sign me up.

Around this same time in my life, I had people asking me questions about what happened to me. If I had the time, I would tell people everything that you have read about me. If I didn't have the time for the whole story, they would get some short anecdotes. The point being, I was telling this story to a lot of people and I began to get a continued response:

*That's crazy...You should write a book.*

# CHAPTER 19

# GRANDMA

———

**CHRISTMAS: 2018**

When I woke up Christmas morning, I wasn't feeling so hot. I took some medicine to try and combat the symptoms before they got too bad. We opened presents, and I was hanging in there. As the afternoon approached, my mom checked in with me to see how I was doing.

"So, you think you can make it to Gram's?" my mom asked, standing in the doorway of my room because I had crawled back into bed.

I sat up and cleared my throat. "I mean," I thought about how I felt for a second, "I feel better than when I woke up. But I also don't want to get people sick."

"How about this: I'll call them and give them the full disclosure. If they don't care, which I highly doubt they will, the decision will be yours."

She exited the room and went to make the phone call to my grandma. My mother's prediction was right, and she relayed me the message. It was up to me. I sat on the edge of my bed wondering to myself if this was going to hold up, or if I was going to have to spend Christmas Day by myself, which was a depressing thought.

"Can we bring medicine in case I start feeling crappy? I don't want to spend Christmas home alone, plus…" I didn't know if it would be rude to say, but my mom beat me to it.

"Yes, I know, your grandparents *are* getting older."

My face looked surprised as she read my mind. "Well yeah, that. I don't want to have any regrets in case, God forbid, something happened."

"Well then suck it up, champ. We'll bring your medicine. You look fine to me; your grandparents want to see you."

So, we suited up to go, and I'm sure glad I did. It was an ugly sweater-themed Christmas party, which was something my grandma had on her bucket list.

My grandma lived for Christmas Day; it was her favorite holiday. She would get all festive with the baking and decorating and spoiling the grandchildren. It was what kept her young, as she put it. My sweater was sky blue with red around the collar and wrists. In the center was a pack of flamingos decked out in Santa hats and Christmas lights, which actually lit up on the sweater. The flamingos were on an island, with the sun shining in the backdrop. I was pretty proud of it.

My grandparents really took the Christmas sweater thing seriously. My grandma had a sweater with an elf peeing on the snow, which for those who know my grandma, this is her in a nutshell. It was a bad or "naughty" sweater in her mind, and she thought it was funny. I got a kick out of it, and so did everyone else. What did Pop have on that could match Gram's spunk? A "Welcome to the North Pole Casino" sweater, with Santa on the front making off with a fat stack of cash.

My grandpa was always the provider for his family and prided himself on his work ethic. Raising four girls and being able to provide for them wasn't an easy task back in the day. Pop had quite the impressive resume although he never boasted about it being the humble man he was. He served in the Navy, worked two jobs his whole life one of them being the Fire Captain in West Orange. On top of that he helped nurse grandma back to health during her years of medical turbulence. He didn't view himself in a grandiose fashion, as he put it, he was doing what was necessary for the ones he loved.

Gram wasn't just all spunk; she was also very knowledgeable when it came to our condition. She was tough as nails also with the will of a thousand men. She was always doing research finding ways to help get closer to a cure. My grandma had a doctor in New Jersey who had a confocal machine. My grandma would go to her and get this scope test done. The doctor who had the machine got a grant to do research in Houston, which is where my grandma went for one of her procedures. The procedures were optional, but my grandma wanted to do it.

What the confocal machine did was look around to see if polyps were turning into adenomas. Adenomas are precancerous bumps that run the risk of turning into cancer and spreading. The machine would release a dye that lights up your stomach and goes seven layers deep into the lining. It would highlight the adenomas if there were any to begin with. The doctor would then go down a separate time to remove any highlighted adenomas. Even though my grandma was doing this optionally, it is something I will have to do in my life eventually.

My grandma didn't necessarily have to do it, but she did for a number of reasons. One, she found this great machine and doctor for us to go to when we need this procedure done. Thankfully, we found another doctor in New Jersey who has the same machine and does the same procedure. Secondly, the adenomas they were removing from her stomach lining were being used for research by this doctor for her research grant. Any way my grandma could contribute to helping, she did—even if it meant traveling, spending money, and sacrificing her body a little bit. She was doing these procedures over the course of five years and had roughly 150 adenomas removed from her stomach that were used for research.

My grandma also loved playing Secret Santa, grab bag style. My grandma started this tradition a couple of years prior to add some spice to the holidays. She wanted it to be "cutthroat," as she put it, because that's the only way it can be a goofy good time. How it's played is that everyone brings a random gift that can be placed in a bag. The bags are put by the tree, with a number on them. Then, we do a raffle of the order you get to pick. Picking first is the worst in this game because everyone going after you can steal your gift. But if someone steals your gift you have a chance to steal it back. Which led to an environment of botched poker faces as people tried to hold onto the gift they actually wanted while pretending they didn't.

My grandma had a keen ability to sniff out who liked what and would take pleasure in stealing the gift to stir the pot if everyone else was being too nice. That mischievous persona she would adopt would never last long, because if she stole from a grandchild the gift they wanted, it would go back to them. And, if they didn't get the gift they wanted, Gram always made sure to sneak you into the kitchen to slip you a hundred-dollar bill when the parents weren't looking. Although on this particular Christmas, she got caught. She whispered to me and snuck me into the kitchen. I smiled because I knew all too well what was coming next.

"Here, this is for you dear." She slipped me a hundred-dollar bill. "This is for your birthday."

I smiled. "You know Mom isn't gonna be happy about this," I said as I tucked the bill into my pocket. You can't say no to Gram.

"I don't care what your mother thinks because I'm her mother. I have seniority," she said in a "gotcha" manner.

My mom, right on cue, sniffed out what was going on.

"What are you doing, Mom?" my mom asked, lecturing grandma as she clearly knew what was going on. Then she turned to direct the blame at me. "And what are you doing? I told you to say no to your grandma."

"Oh, zip it, Marlene. I'm his grandmother; I'm allowed to spoil him. This wasn't his fault. You're overruled."

I shrugged. "Gram makes the rules, not me, Mom."

My mom rolled her eyes. "Haven't you given him enough, Mom?"

"No, not yet. I still have more to give. This ain't your money, honey. I don't see what the problem is."

I flashed a sarcastic smirk. and swung my head toward my mom. "You know, she has a point mom."

"When you're a grandmother, you'll understand it," my grandma said.

My mom's facial expression widened. "Okay, we don't need to rush to that yet."

I laughed, and our kitchen meeting was dismissed. Secret Santa had wrapped up, and Gram was done dispersing her money around to the grandchildren. I was a little under the weather but nothing crazy, I felt good the majority of the time. The memory of us all dressed up in goofy Christmas sweaters, teasing each other with our grab bag stealing, and showering each other in gifts was a great way to bring joy to my holiday. Spending it at home by myself wouldn't have been right. I was glad I ultimately pulled the trigger to go, because little did I know, this would be the last Christmas Day we would have with my grandma.

## CHAPTER 20

# ROUTINE TRAIN WRECK

—

*Life is an endless series of train wrecks with only brief com-mercial-like breaks of happiness."*

—*DEADPOOL*

In February of 2019, that good luck streak was over. We were now back to the routinely scheduled train wreck, and it would be a while before we got back to the happiness. We discovered that my grandma had stage 4 cancer. I remember the day the news was broken to me.

"There is no easy way in saying this to you guys. You're adults, so I'm going to say it." My mom was struggling to tell me and my brother, I could tell something bad was coming. "Grandma...She has cancer."

Immediately after the sentence came out of her mouth, she burst into tears. My heart sank into my stomach. I'd had a feeling it was about Grandma, but I was hoping I was wrong. My brother and I immediately went over and hugged her. We were consoling each other.

"It's going to be okay, guys; we're going to get through this," she kept saying over and over.

I didn't have words; it felt like my world had been rocked. As strange as it sounds, my grandma was immortal in my eyes. I never could picture her dying or getting sick. I'm not sure why this is, but I remember that's how I felt. Everyone dies, it's a part of life, but not for my grandma. Maybe it's because I loved her so much that I didn't want to think of that possibility. Perhaps I'm not the only person who has felt this way. Through the tears I tried to stay optimistic.

"They don't know what it is yet right? She can still fight it...right?"

"We don't know for sure yet. If you know your grandma, you know she's going to fight it. We don't know what the exact diagnosis is yet. We are going to have to get her tested to find out for sure."

During this time, I was at school while we waited. I would check in on grandma and call her multiple times a week. I remember the first time I called her; I was scared. I was never scared to talk to my grandma before. But this time, I didn't think I could be strong on the phone. I was worried I was going to break down crying on the phone. Initially, I delayed the first phone call to Gram and was in denial over the news. I remember my Aunt Maria texting me saying that it's okay to call Gram, that she's strong and she is okay. She told me that it's fine if I cry on the phone and if I'm scared because we all were scared. So, I decided to put my fear to the side and call her.

"Hey, Michael," she emphatically said before I could say hello.

"Hi Gram, how are you doing?" I managed to squeak out, fighting back tears.

"Well, I'm doing alright. There isn't much I can do about it you know?"

"I know…are you okay though?"

"I'm fine. I am. We have to take things one step at a time."

"When do you think they're going to know what it is?"

"Well, we have to get the blood results back to know for sure. We went to go see Dr. Morton for that. Some things came back inconclusive, so they have to retest my blood to see what it is for certain."

"So, they don't know yet? Do they have any good news that we can build off of?"

"Well, Dr. Morton said my blood levels were good, but that doesn't tell us what kind of cancer it is."

"That has to mean something good, right? I mean you feel good, right?"

"Yeah, I feel good. I've felt minor aches over the past couple of weeks prior to me getting checked but that was because of the cancer that we now know of."

"Yeah, but I'm going to try and take it as a good thing. Good blood work and you moving around has to be something good," I kept repeating more for myself than anyone else.

"Oh, you're so sweet, Michael. You always look for the positive. I'm going to be fine; you don't have to worry. You have to focus on school. That is more important. Anyway, how's that book coming along that you were writing?"

Oh man, she remembered from when I told her. My aunt and mom had mentioned it around her as well. I had told my mom I was meeting with one of my professors at Ramapo to work on the book. No one in my family had read it yet, and only my mom, grandma, and aunt knew about it.

"I have some pages written so far; they need some proof-reading and editing."

"Well, if you wouldn't mind, I would love to read them."

I couldn't say no to her. If she wanted to read them, now was the time to get over my fears and to open up to the family, slowly but surely. I knew my grandma wouldn't judge or be offended by anything. I knew if she liked it, it would be a story worth telling. So, after our phone call, I began taking my work more seriously and sending it to her so she could read it.

Later that night, I began typing and editing pages to send to Gram. Once I had ten pages proofread and structured, I emailed them to her. I would start off small, and if it was good, I would continue sending more. Typing ten pages at a time didn't take too long and worked well with my school-work. I sent her a text letting her know I sent it. It was late at night, so I knew she wouldn't read it until the next day. This is what started the process of me getting over my fears and taking my book more seriously.

I continued on with school that week as we were waiting for the definitive results for my grandma. She was nervous; we all were nervous, but we tried to keep ourselves busy. I was trying to keep positive thoughts going and stayed busy with school. After I got back from my classes I received a text from my grandma, "I read the first chapter of your book. You are an unbelievable writer. It is so professional. That's a good field for you. You amaze me. Although I found two typos."

I read the text partially crying and laughed at her mentioning the typos. I appreciated her honesty. My biggest fear with writing the book was I thought I would be airing out my family's dirty laundry, so to speak. The absolute last thing I wanted was to destroy my relationship with my family over writing this book. I needed my family's blessing, but I was too afraid to ask. My grandma gave me her blessing saying how talented I am, and how much she loves what she read.

She wanted me to continue sending her more, which I would continue to do every single week.

My grandma was a huge advocate for polyposis her entire life. She did voluntary procedures to help find a cure for our condition that she didn't have to do. She was always doing this, and she was traveling all over to do it. She often said that she wouldn't be able to die in peace until she gave the blueprint for me, my mom, and my aunt to have a cure for our condition. It was her lifelong goal to make sure that we would be okay for the rest of our lives. When she saw that I was taking initiative to tell our story, her eyes lit up. She loved the idea. She hoped that it would reach a lot of people and save a lot of lives.

After hearing my grandma tried to write about our journey but couldn't do it, I knew that this was my calling in life. She did so much for our condition; I wouldn't be here if it weren't for her work and courage. It's crazy to think about the timeline of my family's history with this condition, one small blip in that and I might not be here. It was only fitting that I continued to do what I know best, which was to continue documenting our story in the hopes that we could save lives and help people who need it.

Needless to say, when my grandmother got her test results back. It was not good news.

---

Strange but beautiful things can be found in an awful situation. The love my grandma received from our whole family during this challenging time was boundless. She was actually taken aback by all the love and support she got. She knew she was loved, but she never in a million years thought she was loved to this extent. I remember her telling me that there was something oddly satisfying about seeing all the love and support she was getting while she was still alive. She made an interesting point to me: that most people only get this love when they are already passed and it's too late. She said that her seeing all the love and support while she was still here gave her some closure on the life that she had lived.

As time went on, Gram, my aunt, and my mom continued reading my book. Each time I sent more to my grandma, it would get more personal and dive deeper into my raw emotions. With each email getting more personal, I always feared I would get negative feedback. I learned through my grandma and my aunt that everything I wrote is something they all felt at one point too. It brought us closer together than we already were, because the emotions that I was writing about is something they could never put into words until now.

The support I got was overwhelming and I still hold onto text messages that my grandma sent to me during the process. My favorite one that eliminated my fears of over expressing myself was as follows:

*"You are the only one who could write this book. You captured all of the emotions and feelings and fear that we all had. You're just amazing and you are an excellent writer. Thank you for doing this. I would really like you to have it published because it is something that would help other people with this disease. Great job."*

My eyes filled up with tears as I looked down into my phone. It was clear to me for a while what my purpose in life was, but this made it stronger. A couple of years ago, I was in denial over my surgery. I never thought I would be able to open up about it with friends and family, let alone write a book. It all started with my grandma and how she built me up when she would take care of me when I was sick.

One weekend I came home from school to help rearrange things in my grandma's house. I helped move a fridge upstairs by her room so she didn't need to walk down the stairs anymore. I moved junk and anything that made it difficult to walk in the basement, helping out with little things that made navigating her house more easily. After the day was over, we ordered takeout for dinner. My grandma had trouble moving around on this day and was staying in bed.

I went up to her room and laid in her bed with her and we ate dinner together. It was me and her, and we began talking. We had an honest heart-to-heart.

"The ribs are good, right, Gram?" I said with a smile, holding her hand, trying to make her feel better.

"I always loved these ribs; they are good." She was holding onto a pink Squishmallow pillow with her other hand while we talked.

"You love this Squishmallow, don't you, Gram?"

"He's my buddy. I love him. I take him with me to chemo."

I was fighting back tears as we talked, trying to be strong for her. I gripped tightly onto her hand.

"How are you feeling, Gram? Just needed more rest today?"

"Well Michael, I'm tired. I don't have the same energy, and I'm a little lightheaded, almost like I'm having a vertigo attack."

"Are you hydrated, Gram? Maybe you're dehydrated; that happens to me when I don't drink enough."

"That could be a possibility. Who knows…I needed to rest today."

"It's okay, Gram. You have earned that right. You don't need to leave bed; that's what I'm here for. That's why I came here today so you can get around easier."

"You're so sweet. I love you. You didn't have to."

"Nonsense, Gram. I would do it every single time."

"Michael, you're an old soul. Do you know that?"

"Wouldn't be the first time someone has said that to me," I chuckled.

"I'm serious. You are not like most people. You are an old soul, and I say that as a compliment. You have a huge heart; you've helped so many people already, and I know you're going to continue to do that. I have no worries about you."

"Thank you, Gram. It means a lot to me. I try my hardest."

"You do a great job, sweetie. Do you remember when I said that God put you here for a special reason—we didn't know why yet? I know now what it is."

"What is it?" I said intrigued.

She propped herself up in bed. "God put you here to save your mom's life. I mean that—your mom wasn't gonna get tested as she got older. She wasn't going to follow up with appointments like me and you would. She only became more open about it after she had you and after she saw how well you handled it."

Many emotions flooded me as I gripped my grandma's hand. I was fighting back tears, and I looked at her. "You mean that?"

"Yes, absolutely. There is no doubt in my mind. You're going to help other people too, and you already have. This is why God put you here. We now know why."

"Thank you, Gram. It means a lot to hear that."

"It's the truth; you're the strongest person I know. Your attitude and how positive you are is something that is a gift."

"Well, I wasn't always positive, Gram—you know that. I would have to respectfully disagree; you are the strongest person I've ever met. I could never be where I am if I didn't learn from you."

"None of us were positive during our recovery process, but the way you overcame it is a gift. I always tell people that you're the strongest person I know."

"C'mon Gram, don't sell yourself short. I respect that you think that of me, but I still have to say you're the strongest person I have ever met."

"What did I do to deserve that title? I'm being honest."

"Gram, do I have to read you a list of the things you have overcome? You lost your mom at seventeen to a strange disease no one knew about. Then you found out you had this condition, and you were basically a guinea pig for five years. They did all those experimental tests and surgeries on you. Then you had four daughters, two of whom have this issue and you nursed them back to health. Then it was my turn, and you nursed me back to health. It's not a comparison, your strength and what you endured is the reason my life is so great today."

My grandma sat there and nodded as if she didn't realize all of the things she accomplished. She was always so busy helping and giving her time to others that she had forgotten all that she achieved. That is a testament to the character of her heart, which was so pure.

After we were done eating, I walked into the bathroom. I sat on the edge of the bath and stared into my hands wondering how life would ever be okay without my Gram. The tears started and didn't stop for what seemed like an eternity. I wasn't ready to accept that this was real. These tears, though, were good tears, if that makes any sense. What she told me that day I will never forget. I will hold onto those words and that memory dearly. Her words to me are the motivation I still use to this day whenever I begin to feel down. Her words are what I consistently use to drown out the outsider, whenever it rears its ugly head.

## CHAPTER 21

# FULL CIRCLE

———

My grandma was an unbelievably strong person who knew her body well. I can't stress it enough: my grandma during her last days was the strongest person I ever knew. I genuinely mean it. I will admire her for the rest of my life. She understood the grief losing her was going to cause the family, and she made it as easy as humanly possible given the circumstances she was dealt.

It was a Thursday morning as I prepared to go to class. I was brushing my teeth and I noticed I was getting a phone call from my brother. A phone call from my brother meant bad news was probably coming. I stared at the phone as it was on the kitchen sink vibrating. My roommates were awake, getting ready for class like I was. I closed my eyes, grabbed the phone, and answered.

"What's up?" I asked with my eyes closed waiting for the bomb to drop.

"It's Grandma." He paused. "Mom thinks she isn't going to make it past today." He began to cry, which was rare for my brother to do. He slowly composed himself. "I'm gonna pick you up, okay? Mom wants us all at the hospital so cancel your class today if you have one."

After he said she was expecting to pass, my world stopped for a moment. How was it, after today, that my grandma would not be here anymore? No more birthday text messages, no more Christmas Day shenanigans, no more club trips... Tears poured out of my eyes as if they were faucets. My cheeks glistened as they started to drip on my phone too. I wiped the tears off my phone, sniffled, and responded, "Okay...let me know when you're coming. I need a second."

I hung up, and the pain started to hit me. I was crying, sobbing in the hallway of my apartment. The thought of losing my grandma hurt so deeply I didn't know if I was ever going to stop crying, let alone hold it together in front of my roommates. How was I going to be able to hold it together in front of my grandma and my family? As I sat in the hall crying, I pulled out my phone to let my professors know I wasn't going to be around. My roommate heard me crying and came out into the hallway to check up on me.

"Hey man, is everything alright?"

I sat wiping my eyes and blowing my nose. "They don't think my grandma..." I choked up trying to get the words out. "They don't think she's gonna make it past the day." The tears cascaded down my face once again. I've never cried like that before in my life; the pain was so deep. In a way, it felt like I was being told a part of me was dying.

My roommate stood there trying to understand the pain I was in. "I'm so sorry to hear, man. I've been through it too with my grandparents, and I want you to know I'm here for you, bro."

I nodded my head. "I know. It's too hard right now. Today is going to be a tough day."

He understood, and he assumed when I came back that night the news wasn't going to be good. I was so nervous about being vulnerable in front of my roommates, which was stupid because they were incredibly understanding, and they let me cry the day away.

## LAST DAY

My brother picked me up, and we began the somber car ride to the hospital. There wasn't much to say besides how much the situation sucks. Typically, my brother and I would talk sports or current events on drives like this, but sugarcoating this time didn't feel right. We sat, eyes red and dry from crying, and prepared for more emotional outbursts.

When we arrived, the greeting with my family was obviously heart-wrenching and extremely difficult. We were all sad and knew what was going on. My grandma looked good for what was the final day I saw her. She looked like normal Gram for the most part. She sat propped up in the bed, her bruised arms sat crossed across her stomach. When I walked in, she greeted me sitting upright. I said hello to the rest of my family who were hiding expressions of grief the best they could. I tried as well.

My grandma wanted me to sit by her, and I held her hand. She told story after story in front of all of us. She was putting on a show for us. My mom was convinced earlier that morning her time was coming. The cancer was progressing, and she had a detailed vision of heaven that day. My mom said she was describing a bridge with a beautiful river flowing underneath it. On the bridge were her loved ones, who she had missed. Her mom, cousins, friends, her sister, and Dr. Gelernt who was her surgeon whom she loved dearly. When she woke up and described this detailed vision to my mom and my aunt, they both decided time was probably running out.

This was a smart assumption, except the grandma in the room that day didn't seem like she was dying. She was still telling us funny stories from her life, which we enjoyed so much. Although, truth be told, I wasn't listening to what she was saying because I was too focused on not totally losing it and bursting into tears. I could barely make out what she was saying because I was studying her every move and gesture trying to etch her essence into my brain knowing we were on borrowed time. I tried to ignore the reality that this story time she was sharing with us was going to be the last.

The visit wasn't as bad as I thought initially; it was because my grandma made it easy for us. It was like she wasn't in pain, and if she was, she wasn't showing it to us. Perhaps she put on a show and a brave face, and if she did then I respect her more. Her bravery and strength in the face of cancer was so admirable. Her belief in a life after this one was also so strong; she didn't have fear in her final moments, which made me believe more in what she tried to tell me most of her life. *I sure hope she's right.*

My grandma managed to hold on for one last night. I was emotionally drained and had a final the following morning. After my final, as I was heading back to my apartment, my phone began to buzz again. This time from my mom.

I knew what the news was going to be.

"Hello?" I answered, my head facing the floor and eyes closed.

"Hey sweetie, Grandma is…she's going to pass soon." She paused briefly. "But we have you on speaker phone if you want to say anything to her. She can hear you, but her voice is weak. I can tell you what she's mouthing if you want."

I wasn't expecting this, and I began to tear up. I was about to say the final words to my grandma.

"I love you, Gram. I love you so much...." My voice began to quiver uncontrollably.

"She's mouthing back clearly, 'I love you too,' and she lit up when you said that," my mom said happily.

"Tell her I'm going to write the book like she wanted, and I'm going to continue to get checked,"

"She's emphatically nodding her head on that one, Michael."

"And...I'm going to make you proud...and I'm going to miss you...so much."

The call was over. Those were my last words to my Gram. I sat on the couch in my apartment, tears flowing down my face and onto the floor in a puddle beneath me. I was crushed.

## AFTERSHOCK

My grandma's wake and funeral were extremely moving. My grandma, the stylish diva she was, was buried in a rose gold casket. Every person who came to pay their respects was astonished at the casket. That was Gram, always going out in style. The wake was overwhelming as the line was non-stop with people coming all day long without a break. It was endless, and I was overwhelmed and tired from standing beside her beautiful casket. Person after person came up saying how great of a woman my grandma was. A fair amount of the people seemed to have known me, and the other grandchildren as she would brag about us each constantly. She did live for her grandchildren.

After the loss of my grandma, the time that followed was not easy. It was especially difficult for my grandpa, who lost the love of his life and his soulmate. If I was hurting, imagine how he was hurting? So, I pitched in as much as I could, along with the rest of my family, to spend as much time with

Pop as possible. During the time when I didn't have class or work, I gave my time to my grandpa, which I'm glad I did because our mutual grief brought us closer than ever. We were always close before, but my grandma was the talker. She would yap on the phone with the grandchildren and her daughters for hours. Pop would get the phone from her for a good five minutes; that's all he needed and then he went back to watching the tube. Pop didn't have any fancy technology; an old flip phone was all he needed.

Alongside navigating my Pop's grief, my mom had to get her endoscope tests done. She had to do it for two reasons. Firstly, she promised my grandma as a dying wish she would get it done. And secondly, she couldn't give up on me considering how I had handled my situation. It was a good thing she got her scopes done because we unfortunately didn't get great news. It turned out my mom had polyps because they still left a small portion of her large intestine behind.

My mom's medical history is complicated, so much so my surgeons didn't know what they did to her back in the day. They were totally unaware she had any of her large intestine left. Back when my mom was sick in the 1980s, she didn't want to get a stoma, so she waited until something better came along. She waited until after college, and she started to get sick. The polyps began to cause issues in her digestive tract, and time was running out. Her surgeons made this clear to her and told her the Koch Pouch was the only option.

My mom didn't want a reservoir of any kind, but the doctors had to do something to save her life. So, they did, and the extent to what was done isn't entirely known. What we did know was a small portion of the large intestine was left behind, and it had to get removed soon! It seemed she had some of her rectum left intact, similar to what was done to my Aunt Ronnie and my grandma, which I touched on earlier. We were lucky we caught it when we did. It seemed like things were now beginning to snowball in the wrong direction again. We lost Grandma, the leader of the club, and now my mom had to get operated on.

Dr. Gorfine was out of the office for medical reasons, so he referred us to his understudy Dr. Chessin. Not only were we without Gram, but now we were without Dr. Gorfine too. I know Dr. Chessin is his guy, but still not having Dr. G on the case was another stress we didn't need. They told us they were going to reverse what my mom had, to having a J-pouch like me and my aunt. This concerned me for a number of reasons because I understood the logistics behind what they were doing. Five years ago, I was told J-pouches were a non-reversible surgery. Five years later, we're being told that not only can it be done, but it can be done laparoscopy.

I had trouble believing some of this at first, especially with how easy they made it sound. I began to shake that thought off because then I realized my mom was going to have to live with the bag again for a brief period of time. This news was a blow because I understood how much of a process this was going to be. It was going to be three surgeries, three recoveries spread out over the course of a year. Along with that, my mom was going to have to live with a bag, which is something she swore she would never do again. I was worried this was going to be too much for her to handle. I know she had a promise to fulfill but I knew how tough this was going to be and I naturally worried.

It was a process indeed; my mom had a surgery in September that got complicated. She had to spend a week in the ICU. Then after she got on her feet from that operation to remove a small polyp, which was supposed to be an overnighter, it was time for the big one. Even the small, easy surgery was difficult this time around.

Then came the big, reversal surgery, which was six hours long. I'll never forget the gut-wrenching angst I felt that day as I tried to not look at the clock. Trying desperately to distract myself anyway I could, until the day continued to drag on without a call from my dad. It was a little over six hours, when I began to panic. *This must be how my mother felt when I was under the knife.* Then right as I was beginning to slip deeper into a darker place mentally, the phone rang.

*Bzzz... Bzzz... Bzzz...*

I stared at the phone, and flinchingly reached to pick it up. "Hello?"

"Dr. Chessin did a beautiful job, everything mother wanted. He did a laparoscopy, so Mommy doesn't have any new scars. The incision is nothing—barely noticeable."

I mouthed "thank God" to myself as I closed my eyes. "Beautiful. I was praying for this to be the outcome we would have."

"Yup, she's all good. Couldn't have gone any better. I'm so glad this is over because this isn't easy on me either, ya know."

"I know, Dad. I know."

"Sitting here for hours for your surgeries, wondering if you were going to be okay. I know you guys are the club, but I think I might deserve an honorary membership to it too."

I never considered my dad not a part of the club; it was never meant to be like that. It was only created to help me feel like less of an outcast. For all of us, being that we live with this rare disease. But my dad, along with my brother, grandpa, and all the other family members who constantly did favors for me were a part of the club. In a different way, I wanted to make that clear to him. I can't imagine it from his perspective. I was a nervous wreck for my mom's operations, but I was away at school. My dad was at the hospital, watching the doctors come in and out of the OR to give him updates in blood covered scrubs. It wasn't like my dad had only done this once. He did it thirty years ago with my mom, then he did it with my aunt and me, now back again to my mom. He needed to feel as important as the rest of us. He may not have had the condition, but he sure was impacted by it.

"Of course, you are, Pops, and you know it isn't like that."

He was fighting tears; it was an emotional day—an emotional year, for that matter. "I know it isn't," he said, sniffling. "I want to be included too, that's all."

I would come home whenever I could on weekends to visit my mom. I would call and check on her throughout the days when I could. I was concerned about my mom's mental well-being after the physical aspect was looking more positive. Much to my surprise, my mom handled it and handled it far better than I had expected. I thought she was going to be mad and resentful over the bag, but instead she had the same "shit happens" attitude I had in the hospital. She knew it was only temporary, and she was going to handle it and get through it.

The roles had suddenly reversed. Years ago, my mom was the one worrying frantically over my well-being, while I was the subject of the operations. Now, I was the one worrying over my mom's well-being as she was the subject in question. I got to see the impact of my own attitude from a third-party perspective in a way. I was so worried and anxious about my mom leading up to the surgery, during, and after that when I saw her taking the challenge head on in good faith it allowed me to exhale. She showed me she was going to be fine, and while I naturally still worried like I'm sure she did with me, it made it a hell of a lot easier. This attitude my mom was showing was something she swore she could never adopt. My mom has admitted to me she isn't sure what life would be like if I didn't handle things the way I did and if things didn't unfold the way they did. All I know is, I'm glad we'll never have to find out.

Seeing her handle the situation so gracefully made me realize life had come full circle. I saw that how I handled our ever-evolving condition changed my mom's overall view, which is something that was necessary to happen in order for her to be here today.

I'm here today because my grandma never gave up back in the day after losing her mom at such a young age. Even after her and her sister endured hell from their condition. All of this was decades of perseverance by my grandma, her sister, my grandpa, my aunt, and my mom. One blip in the time-line, and the reality that I'm not here becomes more likely. It's crazy how some things work out mysteriously perfect. *Is this another example of fate?*

My mom handled her time with the bag better than I did, and it was time for her to be reconnected onto a life of good health. Except when you're a Caprio, plot twists are always interjected to spice things up. My mom was fortunate enough (sarcasm) to be in the hospital as the coronavirus pandemic struck New York City and the United States. On one hand, my mom was having a happy day because she was being reconnected and the bag was going to be gone forever this time. But on the other hand, she had to be rushed out early in scary fashion. I was sitting at home on my couch watching the president give updates to Americans as the case numbers began to rise. They were talking about rushing in the Army CORE of engineers to build makeshift hospitals. All they kept saying on the news was that the weak and vulnerable were the most at risk. And I had my mom cooped up in Mount Sinai, the epicenter of the current outbreak recovering from a surgery. I kept thinking to myself, *Please God, after all we have been through, get her home safely.*

Luckily, God or someone was on our side and did get her home safely. *Perhaps it was Gram; it would have been sick and cruel for us to endure all that to have her get Covid on the cusp of her final recovery.* I completely sterilized the entire house prior to her arrival to make sure the coronavirus was not present. My mom was brought home by my aunt, and we were able to get her set up safely. My surgeon had rushed my mom out of the hospital and the way she described it to me was quite terrifying.

She said he and all the other doctors were in full Hazmat suits, and people were cleaning the hallways with industrial like cleaners while frantically moving patients out of the hospital preparing for a surge of sick patients. It was something out of the movie *Outbreak*, except my mom said this was no movie which made it a moment she would never forget the rest of her life. Because she was rushed out early, the drama didn't end for us. She had a drain in her which was draining an abscess. Under normal circumstances she would've stayed until it was time to take it out. Under Covid circumstances, she had to go home with that drain until further notice. So, I had to play the role of nurse until our surgeons in the city were able to get us an appointment to get the damned thing removed. Which didn't happen for weeks because the hospital offices weren't in use, and our surgeons were working as overflow doctors in Covid wards.

I didn't mind playing the role of nurse since she had done it so many times for me. I was so happy to have her home safe and sound. I wanted her out of the city to stay away from catching the virus because in her current state I feared she wouldn't be able to beat it. I'm thankful and blessed she wasn't one of the people to get sick in the beginning. I think that was Gram pulling strings from above to make sure we were all safe.

# CHAPTER 22

# LIFE GOES ON

———

When the coronavirus locked the country down in March, another hurdle was thrown our way. Not just for my family, but for everyone in the world. In this instance, it was a deadly virus and dealing with the effects of it. An event that happens once in a lifetime—an event that hasn't happened since the Spanish Flu.

My grandpa had been dealing with the loss of my grandma the best he could. We showered him with visits and love. We tried to occupy his mind as much as possible since he had just lost his job due to the Covid lockdowns, which was devastating to him. My grandpa lost everything meaningful in his life in the blink of an eye.

During the initial craziness of the pandemic, my aunt and my grandpa isolated away from everyone. My grandpa is old, and we didn't want him getting the virus. Come May, we eased into having him visit us on Sundays, staying vigilant to keep our quarantine family bubble. When he would visit, we would sit on the couch and watch TV. He was always very comfortable around me, and we were both still grieving the loss of Gram. He would tell me honestly what was going on in his mind. I understood explicitly his thoughts when he told me one day that it felt now like he was just waiting around to die.

That answer hurt me, seeing Pop on the couch stuck in his own head. It was sad. I remembered how that felt for me on some of my worst days after my surgery. I wanted to do anything I could to help him feel less pain. Before Covid happened, when I was on winter break during January of 2020, Pop and I would go to the Sands Casino in Pennsylvania on Wednesdays. Wednesdays were senior's day, and I had nothing going on, so it was a date. On the way up in the car, Pop would always prepare me for the future—a talk I never liked having with him, but we would have it anyways.

"I just want you to know, bud, that your grandma is proud of you, like I am."

I looked over at him as he was driving. "I know, Pop. I know."

"I'm just saying this because I want you to know this now, so that when I'm gone you don't have to wonder. I leave a legacy behind with you, with my grandchildren. I want to make sure the next generation is set up well."

"I know, Pop. I hold onto the lessons you and Gram taught me."

"I know you do. If anything, I hope this last year has taught you how important family is, and if you live a good life, you can make a difference." He composed himself and cried just a little. For my grandpa, this was a huge step toward being open. He wasn't the type to talk about his emotions or anything that would make him cry. "I still can't get over the support your grandmother got at her funeral," he continued.

"She was loved, Pop, and so are you." I had to make that abundantly clear since it seemed he forget this sometimes. I get it though—he was grieving. It's hard to see your worth when you are in such pain.

"I know, bud. I know," he said softly. "Continue to work hard, be there for your cousins and family, and be close with your brother. You guys have a good relationship, that's important." My grandpa made this point clear because of how close he and his brother were. He would get lunch with my Uncle Dave every week, and seeing his brother helped his grief.

"I will, Pop. You know that."

We continued with our drive and arrived at the Sands. We dropped the car off at valet and walked inside. My grandpa was happy to be out and was small talking with everyone he could, including the coat lady, whom he would always flirt with in his goofy Pop way every Wednesday when we would go.

He would take me to his favorite slot machines and would teach me the little tricks he learned throughout the years to pick the right slot machine. Pop's tricks that day worked out well, as we both hit it relatively big. I won $150, and he won $200. If you've learned anything about my grandparents, this meant he was going to be buying lunch and spoiling me a little bit. He was just more subtle about it than my grandma.

After lunch we went to Tommy Hilfiger, and I picked out a nice pair of new shoes. They were about a hundred bucks, which Pop spotted me on.

"I'll take care of this one, bud," he said, wiping my hand away from the cashier.

I looked confused. "This is free money, Pop. I can cover it."

"Use that money for something else over break—food, going out with your buddies, I don't care. I got it this time." He smiled. "Just don't tell your mother."

I laughed; he learned that lesson from Gram.

All the Wednesdays we came, this was the only day we won a nice sum of money. Every Wednesday was enjoyable, but this one was a little better because we had some rewards to our gambling. Above all, it meant the world to my grandpa, which I learned during our conversations in the car.

"I got some stuff at the house that doesn't fit me anymore. It can be yours for when I go to the big firehouse in the sky one day."

I rolled my eyes. "Let's not rush that, Pop. I still enjoy having you around."

He nodded. "I know, but it's going to happen one day, and I want you to be prepared." He got ready to transition to another thought. "You know, that's going to be the happiest day of my life. Not because I don't love you guys but it's because I'll be reunited with your grandmother."

I tried not to get emotional. "I know that, Pop. Still doesn't take away that it will hurt. It already hurt losing Gram."

"But it's the way life is supposed to go; your grandmother and I were never supposed to burry a child or grandchild. Thank God we never did. You…you still have so much life to live. You don't even realize it, bud; this is just the beginning."

"I know." I didn't know what else to say. "I know," I repeated.

"I've lived a good life too, and I know I still have some things to handle here on Earth. I just don't want you to not live your life because of me and your grandmother. You're going to be a writer; you have all these things to look forward to. Just try to remember that."

"I will, Pop, and I know you have. Let's change the subject because we still have time left."

And we did have some time left, but not a lot. My grandparents could've lived to a hundred and it would've still been too soon for me. That's just how it was always going to be. Even though the year without Grandma for Pop was tough, we still had a ton of great memories I'll always hold onto, like our Wednesday senior day trip to the Sands, or every Sunday when he would come over and hang out by our pool during the summer. Especially during the corona summer since activities were limited, we at least had a pool to keep us occupied. When the beaches opened up, we took day trips to the beach.

Pop was starting to have more good moments than bad, even though he was still very much hurting. But, like grandma when she was sick, he saw how loved he was before he passed. The whole family making efforts to be with him is what kept him alive that last year. It even hit a peak on a hot summer in July, where Pop decided to jump into the pool, which he rarely did. Then after a long day in the sun, we spoiled him with his favorite dinner: hot dogs. On his way out of the house that night, he declared that was his best Sunday yet.

That same week, Pop had a stroke. He spent the rest of July and the beginning of August fighting. He gave it his all, but he missed his wife. He made it explicitly clear that this was going to be the happiest day of his life, which it probably was. *I hope. I hope he was with Gram again.* Down here, on Earth, I was destroyed all over again. Just like with Gram, the tears couldn't stop for weeks. I was now without both of my grandparents, and I began a weird transition. It is still a weird transition as I sit here writing this.

Pop got the send-off he wanted; I'm sure him and Gram were smiling from heaven. He had a true fireman's wake, with them keeping guard by his coffin. Captain McGraw decorated the inside of his coffin, and bagpipes were played at his funeral. Holding his casket while walking past service men and women with bagpipes playing in the background was one of the most emotionally chilling moments of my life. But I know he was happy; it was what he wanted.

When we arrived at the cemetery, he was greeted with "Anchors Away" being played by Navy officers. They even did the ceremony where they fold the flag, and they gave it to my aunt. The fireman at the funeral home worked with my grandpa and saw the Navy tattoo on his arm. A tattoo my grandpa hated and regretted getting his whole life was the indicator that made his fireman buddy get in contact with the Navy. He did this on his own, without us telling him. Another lovely surprise to the most moving service I have ever attended, which was only fitting for the best man I ever knew, my grandpa.

After my grandpa passed, we were all looking for signs again. Signs that Gram and Pop were reunited in heaven and that everything was good, something to ease our pain down here, to know they were alright up there. My aunt saw a beautiful double rainbow the day after the service in her neighborhood and took a picture of it. Double rainbows are rare, and in my aunt's head, this was a sign.

A couple of months later, we all continued with our promises of living our lives. I continued to write and work hard at school, which is what they both wanted. My aunt continued back toward changing her career and resumed studying hard for school as well. But the little signs weren't quite doing it for my aunt, so she sought a psychic medium at one point. Truthfully, I could have used a sign myself as I hadn't gotten one in a while so I headed over to her house one night under the pretense of a project I needed help with, but then asked her about the psychic.

I was wearing the shoes Pop had gotten me that day at the casino. I strapped on his favorite gold watch, which I usually wear whenever I get the chance—I like having a piece of him with me. For Gram, I have sentimental items but nothing I can wear, and for obvious reasons. So, I took advantage of being able to wear Pop's gifts, especially since he made it abundantly clear when he was alive that he wanted me to have them when he was gone.

After she helped me with some work, we sat down to have dinner. "So, I went to the psychic this week. Did I tell you what happened yet?" she asked, sticking her fork into her salad.

I finished chewing the pasta in my mouth and swallowed. "I think so, but I'm not sure. I think mom told me a little bit."

"Well, I first asked the psychic if they sent me any signs recently. I didn't tell them the rainbow specifically because I want to make sure this is real."

I stopped eating. "She mentioned the rainbow?"

My aunt smiled. "I asked if they sent a sign, and the lady started to make a high arching motion with her hand that resembled a rainbow. She said that she's hearing something about a rainbow."

I stopped and was shocked. How could she know about the rainbow? My aunt didn't give it away. How could this lady possibly know that if she was faking?

"Wow."

My aunt continued, "That wasn't it. I still had more questions. So, I asked about if there's anything in the closet that I need to know about since I'm stressing about cleaning it out and not throwing away something I need."

"What else do you need?"

"Gram and Pop had money lying around up there as backup cash. It was emergency cash that Pop and Gram hid from us. I have no clue where it is, so I asked about that and guess what?"

"What?" I replied with increasing interest.

"The psychic was saying that she was hearing something about pockets, one of Pop's pockets, and the women was saying she could hear grandma laughing. So, after I heard that, it clicked for me where I had to search. When I got back, I searched in the pockets of Pop's old pants and sure enough, there it was. Three thousand dollars in the pocket of a pair of his pants."

I was always in awe when I got signs from my grandparents, but this was another big one for me. How could a psychic fake those things? Even if they scam or aren't legitimate, how could they know about the pant pockets having money in it in my grandpa's closet. How could they know about the double rainbow? I sat at the table trying to debunk it in my head, but after a little bit I stopped fighting it.

"Wow. That's...that's real."

"Yup kiddo, it's real. They are happy together again. I have no doubts in my mind."

"I'm not going to lie; I was having a little bit of doubt. I needed a sign, and this was the sign I needed," I said smiling.

She finished telling me her psychic stories over dinner. After we were done, I hung out for a little, and then it was time to depart. I sat in my car and looked at Pop's watch sitting on my wrist. I let out a smile. "Thank you guys. I needed that one," I said out loud in the privacy of my car, as if they were with me.

I looked back over at Gram and Pop's house, where they were no longer occupants. Before the sadness could fill my heart again, a wave of reassurance came over me. I remembered the story I just got from Aunt Re—*that was my sign.* They were reunited again, sharing one heart, like they always did. And, I had to hold true on my promise. The promise to continue living my life. And the promise to finish writing this story, which I know for sure they helped me write with guidance from above. As I pulled out of the driveway and down the street, it was time for life to go on. Not to forget Gram and Pop, but to honor them, to make them happy as they look down on me, and to continue making them proud.

I turned right, heading for home when I notice two dimes sitting square in the middle of the empty passenger seat next to me.

I smile, and my heart filled with love.

# ACKNOWLEDGMENTS

---

If you have made it to this point in the book, it means you have read the entirety of my story. First and foremost, thank you to *you,* the reader, for taking the time to experience my journey.

I must start by thanking my family for their unconditional love and support throughout the entirety of my health issues. Pops, thank you for staying calm through the most turbulent of times. You always drove me to every doctor appointment and every operation. I know the long hours waiting in between surgeries was tough and seeing me and Mom at our weakest couldn't have been easy. Thank you for never folding when we needed you to stay strong.

Mom, thank you for never leaving my side at the hospital when I was at my weakest. You slept in a chair by my side every night, and never let me feel alone when I was convinced the world around me was crumbling. You went above and beyond the call of duty for me, and I'll never be able to repay you for what you did.

To my brother, Nicholas, thank you for always being open and understanding when it comes to our condition. You never felt slighted when Mom and Dad had to devote more time and attention to me when I was sick. You have always been a trusted friend and the best brother.

This book wouldn't have been possible without the relationships I had with my grandparents, Juanita and Donald McGraw. Thank you, Gram, for your unconditional love and always being there for all of your grandchildren. You were like our second mother and our best friend. You built me up when I was at my weakest. Your strength and charismatic attitude that you lived your life with has been forever rubbed off on me.

Pop, you were the gold standard of "hard work pays off." You spent your whole life working and never boasted once about your impressive resume. You taught me humility, work ethic, and, most importantly, how to care for the ones you love most. You two were the gold standard of good morals and how to overcome adversity with compassion. It pains me that you couldn't be here with me physically for this moment, but I know for sure you were both pulling strings from above.

Thank you to Maria McGraw, my aunt, for always being there for me. You have always spoiled me with love and your awesome brownie pies.

Thank you to my cousins, "the grandchildren," and "the kids' table" at Christmas and Thanksgiving. We are no longer children anymore, but we have all grown up into men and women Pop and Gram would be proud of. Christopher, Casie, Jessica, Becky, thank you for always staying in touch and being supportive of my dream to write this book. I love you guys.

To all my aunts, uncles, and extended family, thank you for all your overwhelming support during my pre-sale campaign, as well as the entirety of my life. I'm beyond blessed and fortunate to have such a large, loving, and supportive family. There are too many people to name in this section, but your names will be included in the pre-sale contributors.

Dr. Gorfine, thank you for saving my life and giving me the gift of quality of life. You brought me back to health not only with your gifted hands, but also with your compassionate manner. Your humor and lighthearted nature made it a whole lot easier for an eighteen-year-old kid who was scared out of his wits. You are the benchmark for your profession, thank you. I am forever in your debt.

To the nurses and staff at Mount Sinai Hospital in Manhattan, thank you for all your help in bringing me back to a life of health. There is a reason you're regarded as one of the best hospitals in the country; it's well deserved.

To all of my friends who have been by my side from the beginning to now, it's been quite a journey. Thank you for sticking with me through the highs and lows.

Thank you to Eric Koester, Brian Bies, and the team at New Degree Press. Eric you turned my dream into a reality; thank you for giving me this chance. I'm forever thankful for the opportunity you gave me. Brian, thank you for your constant dedication in the publishing process and for helping all the authors out. To everyone who has been working tirelessly behind the scenes at New Degree Press helping authors' dreams become a reality, thank you for your incredible work. You don't get the same attention most of you deserve, but I'm grateful for all of you. Even the ones I haven't met who have been working silently behind the scenes on my cover, layout, and style. This isn't possible without the beautiful work you ladies and gentlemen do.

A huge thank you to my editors Karina Agbisit and Julie Colvin for turning my book into the best it could possibly be. Thank you, Karina, for always encouraging me to expand more in certain areas and offering your two cents. Julie, this book wouldn't be possible without your guidance and understanding of my vision for this book. Our conversations are always productive and enjoyable, and working with you has been a great pleasure. You are just as much a good friend, as well as a talented editor/author.

Finally, thank you to everyone who has believed in me and has supported my writing. You have given me the confidence and support necessary for me to embark on this journey. Thank you to everyone who provided early feedback on my manuscript. I'm thankful for all of your help to make this book the best it could be. A special and sincere thank you from the bottom of my heart to everyone who bought a copy or contributed to my presale campaign. Without your support this book wouldn't be a reality, and it was heartwarming to see the amount of support I received. Thank you to the following:

Susan Hill, Greg Sanger, Aldo Caprio, Geoff Schiffenhaus, Dalton Delrosso, Jordan Yaros, Joanne Walker, Alessandro Kiraly, Judy Rivera, Jessica Modrow, William Metzger, Cassandra Tutalo, Eric Koester, Joanne Lutz, Michael Fiore, Dana Gianfrancesco, Anthony Riebel, Donna Pecci, Irene Hedden, Paula Kiser, Marie McGraw, Brian Garland, Kirsten Micco, Cory Tillery, Mary E. Barrows, Sharron Bello, Marion Campell, Ryan Slater, Khalen Dietz, Nicholas Caprio, Amanda Villano, Amber Allen, Rebecca Berman, Michelle Tutalo, Frances and Anthony Bianchi, Linda and Gary Caddell, Ellen Shapiro, Brian Cawley, Kristina Mancini, Mario Mancini, Linda Mancini, Mark De Mattheis, Pam Bono, Don Bilby, Charles Gamarekian, Maria Scumaci, Marc Parlavecchio, Emmanuel Quianoo, Anthony Mehran, Christine Oaked, Lesley Warren, Rosanna Appio, Michael Dsurney,

Mary McGraw, Avery Miller, Michael Franchino, Dignorach Castillo, Stuart Lasser, Cathy Caprio, Anthony Caprio, James Sullivan, Christopher Marcinek, Stephanie Brumby, Ashely Cavuto, Shelby Smith, Dj Ross, Barry Comerford, Karen Brown, Cynthia Zisis, Arline Oberst, Lucy Gentile, Janice Davey, Maria Shwalb, Joseph Bird, Nancy Filipponi, Rachel Verrone, Veronica Pollock, Robert Mara, James Vilardo, Jesse Farrell, Michael Hyatt, Summer Luciani, Carissa Shook, Alyse Galvin, Marlene Caprio, Nicole Jaronsky, Siisi Quianoo, Alexander Kocovski, Christopher Tutalo, Alyssa Stasse, JP McEvoy, Bridget Darcy, Julian Natelli.

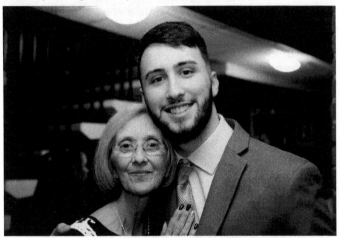

Me and Gram at my grandparents' sixtieth anniversary party.

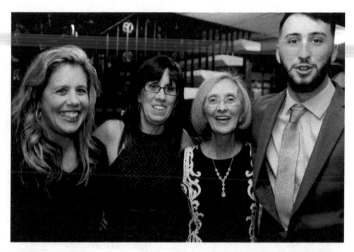

"The Club," me, my grandma, my mom, and my aunt

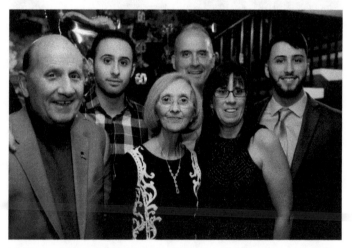

The rest of the gang joins the picture (my brother, my dad, and my grandpa).

# APPENDIX

---

## INTRODUCTION

"Familial Adenomatous Polyposis." Mayo Clinic. Mayo Foundation for Medical Education and Research, December 21, 2018. https://www.mayoclinic.org/diseases-conditions/familial-adenomatous-polyposis/symptoms-causes/syc-20372443.

"Familial Adenomatous Polyposis." NORD (National Organization for Rare Disorders). Accessed January 8, 2021. https://rarediseases.org/rare-diseases/familial-adenomatous-polyposis/.

## CHAPTER 2

Khatri, Minesh. "Ulcerative Colitis Surgery: J-Pouch (IPAA) and Ileostomy Explained." WebMD. January 27, 2020. https://www.webmd.com/ibd-crohns-disease/ulcerative-colitis/uc-surgery#1-2.

## CHAPTER 3

"Familial Adenomatous Polyposis: MedlinePlus Genetics." MedlinePlus. US National Library of Medicine. August 18, 2020. https://medlineplus.gov/genetics/condition/familial-adenomatous-polyposis/.

R, Gedik, and S Müftüoğlu. "Compound Odontoma: Differential Diagnosis and Review of the Literature." *West Indian Medical Journal.* August 20, 2015. https://www.ncbi.nlm.nih.gov/pmc/articles/PMC4668987/.

Pouchitis. Mayo Clinic, Mayo Foundation for Medical Education and Research. September 29, 2020. https://www.mayoclinic.org/diseases-conditions/pouchitis/symptoms-causes/syc-20361991.

## CHAPTER 5

"Caring for Your Jackson-Pratt Drain." Memorial Sloan Kettering Cancer Center. Accessed January 9, 2021. https://www.mskcc.org/cancer-care/patient-education/caring-your-jackson-pratt-drain.

## CHAPTER 8

Anderson, Jenny. "Loneliness Is Bad for Our Health, Now Governments around the World Are Finally Tackling It. Quartz. October 9, 2018." https://qz.com/1413576/loneliness-is-bad-for-our-health-now-governments-around-the-world-are-finally-tackling-the-problem/.

Jones, Carrie M. "The Loneliness Epidemic Revisited: A 2020 Update." CMSWire.com. February 19, 2020. https://www.cmswire.com/digital-workplace/the-loneliness-epidemic-revisited-a-2020-update/.

Lee, Lisa. "NIH Study Probes Impact of Heavy Screen Time on Young Brains." BloombergQuint. December 11, 2018. https://www.bloombergquint.com/technology/screen-time-changes-structure-of-kids-brains-60-minutes-says#gs.ddq1FHk.

Robinson, Lawrence, Melinda Smith, and Jeanne Segal. "Emotional and Psychological Trauma." HelpGuide.org. Accessed February 12, 2021. https://www.helpguide.org/articles/ptsd-trauma/coping-with-emotional-and-psychological-trauma.htm.

Suicide Statistics. National Institute of Mental Health. US Department of Health and Human Services. January 2021. https://www.nimh.nih.gov/health/statistics/suicide.shtml.

Twenge, Jean. "What Might Explain the Current Unhappiness Epidemic?" Ladders. April 23, 2020. https://www.theladders.com/career-advice/what-might-explain-the-current-unhappiness-epidemic.

Tromholt, Morton. "The Facebook Experiment: Quitting Facebook Leads to Higher Levels of Well-Being." Cyberpsychology, behavior and social networking. US National Library of Medicine. November 1, 2016. https://www.liebertpub.com/doi/abs/10.1089/cyber.2016.0259?journalCode=cyber.

## CHAPTER 10

Ghoneim, Mohamed M and Michael W O'Hara. "Depression and Postoperative Complications: an Overview." BMC surgery. BioMed Central. February 2, 2016. https://pubmed.ncbi.nlm. nih.gov/26830195/.


## CHAPTER 11

Saxon, Wolfgang. "Irwin M. Gelernt, 60, Surgeon Specializing in Intestinal Disease." The New York Times. July 4, 1996. https://www.nytimes.com/1996/07/04/nyregion/irwin-m-ge-lernt-60-surgeon-specializing-in-intestinal-disease.html.

Schiller, Don. "The Kock Pouch procedure (Koch Pouch) and other Ileostomy options." KockPouch.com, 2009. http://kockpouch. com/.


## CHAPTER 15

Leuven, Ku. "Mechanism behind Bowel Paralysis after Surgery Revealed." ScienceDaily. June 20, 2017. https://www.science-daily.com/releases/2017/06/170620093143.htm.


## CHAPTER 18

Abrantes, Ana M, et al. "A Pilot Randomized Controlled Trial of Aerobic Exercise as an Adjunct to OCD Treatment. General Hospital Psychiatry 49. November 2017: 51-55." https://pubmed. ncbi.nlm.nih.gov/29122148/.

Allen, Victoria. "Moderate Exercise Just Three Times a Week and Eating Healthy Can Take 10 Years Off Your Brain Age, Study

Says." Daily Mail. December 19, 2018. https://www.dailymail.
co.uk/news/article-6514359/Moderate-exercise-just-three-
times-week-eating-healthy-10-years-brain-age.html.

Amen, Daniel G. MD. *The End of Mental Illness: How Neuroscience is Transforming Psychiatry and Helping Prevent or Reverse
Mood and Anxiety Disorders, ADHD, Addictions, PTSD, Psychosis, Personality Disorders, and More.* Illinois: Tyndale
Momentum, 2020.

Cell Press. "Physical Activity May Leave the Brain More Open
to Change." ScienceDaily. December 7, 2015. https://www.sci-
encedaily.com/releases/2015/12/151207131508.htm.

"Depression and Anxiety: Exercise Eases Symptoms." Mayo Clinic.
Mayo Foundation for Medical Education and Research, September 27, 2017. https://www.mayoclinic.org/diseases-con-
ditions/depression/in-depth/depression-and-exercise/
art-20046495.